LIFE IS MOVEMENT.

We are in perpetual motion. The art is moving thru life skill-fully & mindfully aware of thoughts, feelings and behavior. *Life With Breath* is a journey on discovering the mind/body relationship that is linked through breath. When we lose the relationship with our breath, we lose the connection with our body. It's the same principle with life. The intensity of any given moment is determined by our perception of the moment. As the intensity of the situation rises, so does our perception of pain and/or discomfort. We experience an unpleasant moment, we get lost in the thoughts and emotions triggered by the moment, we lose our relationship with the breath which then diminishes our connection to the body. Typically, our reactions and behaviors don't support our most authentic sense of self and ill-health is the eventual result.

The daily practices in *Life With Breath* serve as a guide and self-care routine to discover YOUR *life with breath*. As you remove your mind from the external environment to the internal environment paying attention only to your breath, the body & mind unite into a self-healing mechanism transform-ing doubt into confidence, fear into courage, hate into love. Discover the wisdom within you. Discover your *life with breath*.

LIFE

with
BREATH

IQ + EQ = NEW YOU

Ed Harrold

For information about this title or to order other books and/or electronic media, contact the publisher:
Go BE Great Inc.
1192 Draper Parkway, #448, Draper, UT 84020
www.edharrold.com
wendy@edharrold.com

Library of Congress Control Number: 2017944341

Print ISBN: 978-0-9990668-3-6
eBook ISBN: 978-0-9990668-9-8
Audio ISBN: 978-0-9990668-7-4

Printed in the United States of America

Cover and Interior design: Kelley Visual and 1106 Design

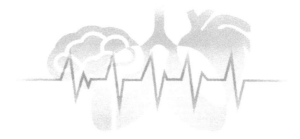

Contents

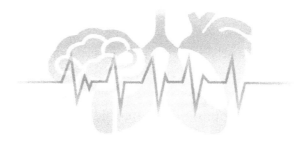

Acknowledgments

THIS BOOK HAS COME TO life thanks to support from family, friends, colleagues, and, above all, you. I want to thank my mother and father, Dorothy and Edward Harrold. They gave me the courage, support, and love to believe I could accomplish anything. They taught me to live without limitations,

I want to thank my lovely and beautiful wife, Wendy, who has supported me throughout my career. She's been my love, my business partner, my best friend, and my confidante. My two precious daughters, Charlotte and Ellen, have taught me humility, patience, and, most of all, love without limitations.

Throughout the journey we call life, there are people who influence us. They mold us in ways we can't comprehend at the time. I want to thank my early competitive sports coaches: Pat Conover, Ray Smith, Steve Merlino, and many others who touched my young mind along the way, refining my skill sets and reminding me to simply be the best you can.

I want to personally thank my friend, coach, and mentor Bill Howarth. Bill was a huge support system in my training and racing in the 22½-mile Around the Island Swim. Above all, Bill was a good friend and was always there for me.

Also, thanks to all the yoga teachers and students I've had the pleasure to work with. And a special thanks to the Kripalu Center for Yoga and Health and senior teachers Yoganand Michael Carroll, Steven Cope, Jonathan Foust, and Larissa Carlson.

Finally, thank you to all the people I'm meeting right now through this book. If you're reading this, you're asking yourself the deeper questions and searching beyond the current model of health, behavior, competition, and our life's purpose/expectations. You're choosing to live beyond the old status quo.

Thank you for pushing me to Go BE Great!

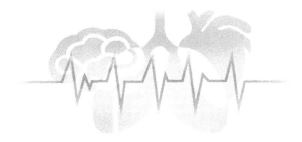

Introduction

FOR AS LONG AS I CAN remember, I've been blessed with the desire to help people. Even as a child, whenever I learned something new, I couldn't wait to teach it to someone else. So coaching and mentoring have always been passions of mine, but it didn't occur to me back then that my passions would turn into my profession.

I grew up in New Jersey on Ventnor Beach. I was raised a hundred yards from the ocean. I excelled in sports, especially water sports, and was known as a "water man." The first thing I'd do every day was look out my bedroom window to see if there were waves. The ocean was my first true love. I feel at home in the water, and the bigger the waves the better. I swim, row, surf, bodysurf, kayak, and sail. Soon after I turned fourteen, I became a beach lifeguard in Ventnor City.

Meanwhile, my parents were grooming me to run the insurance adjusting business they owned, and when I graduated from high school, I followed the plan they'd laid out. By twenty-five, I was running the family business.

In my early thirties, I got married and my wife and I had two beautiful girls together. I had plenty to be grateful for, but I wasn't happy. And the longer I stayed on the course that seemed to work so well for others, the worse I felt. I knew the world was getting darker for me, but I didn't know why. For years I meandered through life, not really feeling connected to a greater power or to nature or even to myself. I thought the critical voice in my head was who I really was, and I was afraid of failure on every level.

By my late thirties, I was unhappy with my career, my marriage was ending, and I was frozen in fear. I was staying out late, drinking too much, eating poorly. I was lost. Or at least I thought I was. Then came the Around the Island Swim.

My Journey to a Life with Breath

In 1994, I competed in the 22½-mile Around the Island Swim in Atlantic City, New Jersey. The only amateur in a field of twenty-seven professional swimmers, I finished fourteenth. This was the turning point for me. I had put my body and mind through my most grueling competitive challenge to date, but as grueling as it was, I was in my element—in my body and in immersed nature.

The Around the Island Swim is a combination ocean and bay marathon at a time of year when the water temperature is fifty-nine degrees on average. Swimmers encounter changes in temperature, tides, and currents. For me, the first seven miles of the race were great. I was swimming effortlessly, without any perceived problems. It was the next ten miles of the race that were truly debilitating and ultimately life-changing. I can't count how many times my mind encouraged me to stop during those ten miles while my body violently revolted against the demands of such a difficult swim. I was vomiting and very cold. I was hallucinating. My body temperature had dropped, and

I was experiencing the early to middle stages of hypothermia. My body and mind were breaking, just like my life seemed to be breaking at the time.

Around mile seventeen, something shifted. Something took over me, or should I say something let go of me—my ego. When the battle within my mind finally seemed to cease, I became empowered. I started to swim like I never had in my life. A warm, bright energy rose from my pelvic basin. It felt like a bottomless source of energy that I had never experienced before. I swam at eighty-five to ninety strokes a minute for the last five and a half miles. Actually, I wasn't swimming anymore—*something greater than me had begun to swim for me, and I was on the ride of my life.*

I didn't want it to end. I felt invincible. I had become one with the water molecules of the ocean in those moments. I wasn't moving my arms against the water like I did when my ego was in charge; the water was now moving my arms. I was in "flow" or "the zone," as the phenomenon is commonly called in athletics. And I never experienced that space again until my introduction to yoga a few years later.

I began my exploration into yoga and yoga breathing as a broken athlete with lower-back and knee injuries sustained from years of individual and team sports. I'd been a competitive athlete in everything from football to surfing since the age of nine, and by my midthirties, I was feeling the effects of overtraining and injury. Not only could I not reach my toes, but also I could barely reach my knees. But damn, I looked good in the mirror!

As an athlete, I wondered why we were never taught the importance of linking breath with movement, or that different breathing techniques facilitate different physiologic functions in the body. I was immediately drawn to the breathing and meditation limbs of yoga as I felt my mind and body reconnecting like they had when I was a child.

We can run from ourselves for only so long. At some point, life catches up with us. In my case, the universe, in all its wisdom, led me to yoga and conscious yoga breathing called pranayama. And that's when I became fully aware of my saboteur, the voice that was stopping me from searching for my true self. For twenty-five years, my saboteur had been at the helm, driving me deep into personal suffering. I didn't know that the power to "BE GREAT" had been inside me all along. When I began practicing mindfulness-based strategies, yoga, pranayama, and meditation, my personal story of transformation began. Through mastering the art of these practices, I learned to overcome my lower ego's need to get attention in ways that devalued my heart and all the goodness afforded me by the universe. I discovered something in myself that raised my self-esteem and led to a new level of self-acceptance. I knew I wasn't perfect, but I noticed that there was some sort of strange perfection to my imperfections. I stopped taking myself so seriously all the time, and I smiled more.

Coming Full Circle

It would have been impossible for me to synthesize the information and create the practices in this book without my inward journey of self-awareness transformation that took place at the Kripalu Center for Yoga and Health in western Massachusetts in the 1990s.

Kripalu is a special place hidden in the mountains of western Massachusetts. The building, an old Jesuit monastery, pulses with energy. There were times early in my training when just walking through those halls made me feel better than I'd ever felt before. The feeling was a relaxed knowing that something bigger than me was coming forth in my personal awareness. I also recall times when I felt scared and incredibly depressed. These feelings, like waves, would wash over me and then new waves would hit, some happy, some sad. Eventually I realized that I was immersed in huge waves of energy and awareness. I just had to surf the waves. Most of surfing is waiting on the board to catch waves. When we choose the wave, it's a better ride than when the wave chooses us.

I won't kid you. It was harder than it sounds. Before studying at Kripalu, my mode of operating was to avoid feeling fear and all other negative emotions at any cost. And believe me, there's a big toll to pay on that road. The price *I* paid was losing the connection with my true self and becoming emotionally numb. My teachers at Kripalu encouraged me to practice the opposite approach, which was to try to feel *everything*. The more I could feel, they explained, the more clear life would become. And as I did this, I began to get new answers to old questions and I began to ask new questions that put me on a path of true self-discovery. For the first time since I was a young child, I began to feel joy and peace and deep love. In essence, I learned to stop censoring my soul.

As I practiced the pranayama breathing techniques combined with the gentle style of yoga taught at Kripalu, I began to truly relax. The breathing and yoga created the neurochemistry for deep relaxation and also told my brain to release hormones that allowed me to see myself differently. In this state of consciousness, I wasn't fully awake, but I also wasn't asleep. I could see through my ego's traps that I would normally fall for. I was a witness in my mind's ear and eye. I could view any old story or imprint without having a knee-jerk reaction or judgment about whether it was bad or good, pain or pleasure. It was relaxing and very exciting all in the same moment!

Over time, these periods of deep meditation led me to see that my greatest fears were hiding my greatest strengths. I could see how each fear had a corresponding strength and that they appeared to be inseparable—one always came with the other. I realized that I'd been telling myself stories that weren't true. When you have the epiphany that one of your stories that fundamentally define you is not true, it triggers the question, "What else do I believe that isn't true?" The state of emotional balance and "beginner's mind" that's produced with pranayama breathing allows us to ask that question, or any question, and receive profound answers.

I subtitled this book *IQ + EQ = New You* because we're designed to always evolve. It's beginner's mind that creates the space for us to grow and evolve as people, as a species, as a family, community, company, and culture. There's a union that takes place between the body and the mind that can happen only through breath. That union makes us more powerful physically, mentally, and emotionally than we could have imagined. In fact, today's research reveals that "flow states" enable us to increase cognitive performance by 500 percent to 700 percent.

I Breathe, Therefore I Am

In yoga, we're concerned with balancing the flow of energy and awareness and raising prana (life force) energy. Pranayama creates this balance by linking the body with the mind. Without the breath, yoga isn't yoga. It's a mindless exercise. When I willfully move my body into asana yoga poses, that's my ego. My ego forces and pushes and cares what I look like in the posture. This is not a union of the body and the mind. This is my ego creating suffering for my mind and body. The breath is what "yokes" the body-mind. It stills the ego, calms the mind, relaxes the body, and guides us safely.

When combined with Western exercise, asana, or any meditative movements, pranayama is one of the highest forms of purification and discipline, as the physical sensation of heat (or tapas) is produced in an effort to purify the body. The longer we stay in the posture, the more detoxifying heat is brought to the surface. As the tapas builds, focusing on the breath keeps us present and provides the space for comfort within the discomfort. In the heat is a deeper awareness of ourselves and our purpose in life. In the heat is the healing.

I discovered that we can apply this same practice of using the breath to remain in a posture to every aspect of our lives. I do this in my own life in an effort to constantly be living the practice of healing. We can practice pranayama in our relationships, our business dealings and decisions, and in sports, hobbies, and other pursuits. The more areas of your life that you bring these breathing practices into, the more balanced and expansive your life will become.

The breath also allows us to ask and explore life's deeper questions without negatively judging others or ourselves. We can use our breath like an archaeologist uses a brush to remove layers of sand and discover old civilizations and stories. The truths of life are buried inside our stories. Conscious breathing empowers us to ask questions and challenge authority in a healthy way on every level of our personal awareness.

There are universal rules everyone can follow—be kind, be patient, be love, be compassion in action—but before we can do these externally, we must do them internally. We see and hear the external world as a direct reflection of how we see and hear ourselves. With this awareness, we can transform ourselves and our lives into the most beautiful expressions of self. It's my breath that saved and transformed my life. My hope is that sharing my experience and practice will do the same for you. My mission is to help you find the same within *you!*

The 30-Day Breath as Medicine program was designed to assist you in healing and transforming as efficiently and effectively as possible, without missing the blind spots. The mindful breathing techniques in this book are designed to restore and repair your biochemical, biomechanical, physiological, and psychological health and well-being. They are self-care tools for shifting the feedback loop of communication with your brain from fight-or-flight response to rest and restore, for retraining the body-mind to operate more often from its parasympathetic system. It's through this system that we strengthen our nervous and cardiovascular systems and allow them to handle more energy without raising our heart rates too high, overloading our bloodstream with high levels of acidity, or increasing inflammation. This will stall the aging process and give you more time to pursue your life's purpose and fulfill your dreams.

You'll learn how to support your overall wellness and cultivate a mindful existence through conscious breathing and the power of breath work. Doing the breathing exercises will help to calm your nervous system, strengthen your cardiovascular system, heighten mental clarity, and improve concentration. The results will include better performance mentally and physically, greater awareness, and the ability to connect with the present moment. Consistent practice induces a sense of centered stillness that makes you more receptive to intuition and spiritual messages. The mission of this book is to help you discover your physical, mental, and emotional greatness. The insights and daily practices in this book will serve as your guide on a magical adventure of healing and transformation.

I'm honored to share this information with you. Enjoy yourself while reading this book, smile deeply inside yourself, and know you're doing something very good for yourself and everyone in your life. And there isn't a rush to finish it—you'll be using these skills for the rest of your life.

GO BE GREAT!

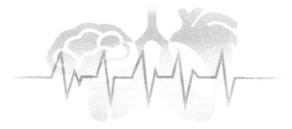

Part One

The Way We Breathe Affects Everything

The Biology of Conscious Breathing

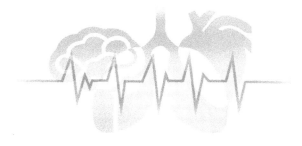

Chapter One

Our Breathing Shapes Our Reality

"Our brain creates our perceptions. Our mind and heart create our values. When we find value in our expanding personal awareness one breath at a time, our perception of ourselves and the world around us evolves."

— ED HARROLD

WE ALL WANT TO FEEL BETTER, have more energy, and be happier, so it's ironic that most people don't know they can fulfill those desires simply and inexpensively. Being healthier, happier, and more energetic is just a breath away. As skeptical as many Westerners can be about Eastern philosophy, it's no surprise that it took decades for our scientific community to comprehend what yogis have known for centuries: *The fastest, easiest way to transform every aspect of our life is through our breathing.*

The way we breathe, fast or slow, mouth open or closed, shallow or deep, directly affects our physiology, psychology, biochemistry, and biomechanics—and it also affects us spiritually. How we think and feel are dramatically affected by how we breathe. By learning and practicing conscious breathing exercises, we can be happier, calmer, and healthier almost immediately.

The ability to manage our emotions and remain calm under pressure has a direct link to professional performance, athletic performance, personal choices, and, ultimately, our health. Whether I'm working with executives or athletes, applying the basic principles and practices in *Life With Breath* produces remarkable results. The improvements have been extraordinary. And just when I think I have it all figured out, the breath, body, and mind teach me something new.

Health, growth, and transformation all begin with our breath. As we move our minds from the external environment to the internal environment, paying attention only to our breath, the body and the mind unite, transforming doubt into confidence, fear into courage, hate into love. Research studies have found that certain breathing practices can reduce the symptoms associated with depression, anxiety, post-traumatic stress disorder, and insomnia.[1]

It All Started with a Simple Breath

It doesn't matter whether you've ever done yoga or pranayama (pronounced: pra-na-ya-ma), also called conscious breathing. Start now by taking a few full, deep breaths, inhaling and exhaling through your nose, and notice how you feel. The thirty-day program in Part Two of this book will share everything you need to know to start and continue your own breathing practice and reap all the physical, mental, and spiritual rewards. This program is the shortcut that took me many years to discover.

When I started learning pranayama, it was to raise energy (prana) levels so I could stay in yoga postures for longer periods of time. I also used pranayama to get into a meditative, reflective mind-set. The breathing practices warmed me up fast and made it easy to settle my monkey mind and create the space for deeper levels of concentration and awareness.

One afternoon, when I should have been on my way to the gym, I was stuck at my desk. By the time I left the office, I had only twenty-five minutes to fit in my workout. On the way to the gym, a voice in my head said, "Ed, remember the breathing techniques you learned and practiced in yoga? Try those in your cardio and weight workouts." When I got to the gym, I started with the lat-pulldown machine and used yogic breathing while I did my ten reps. I completed the set, stood up and felt something I had never felt before. Somehow in that moment, I knew my life would never be the same. There's a lot about that moment that I can't put into words, but physically I felt a lot more heat than I normally felt after doing these reps. The breathing kept my mind locked in on the task at hand. My heart rate went up higher than it normally would and dropped back down to my resting heart rate in just five seconds. I felt amazing. Calm yet excited. That was the turning point. In that moment, I decided to bring pranayama into every aspect of my life and all my training regimens. The results were incredible. That's when I started using what I'd learned with the athletes and executives I coach.

The physiological and psychological aspects of a high-performing executive or business owner are no different from those of an endurance athlete. Both the endurance athlete and the executive need to maintain autonomic balance and encourage fat-burning metabolism all day long. They both need to maintain a balanced mind-set, and when they're at their best, they both operate in the eye of the storm.

As far as I'm concerned, everyone alive is an endurance athlete because life is an endurance event. So we all benefit by lowering our heart rates with high-quality thoughts, feelings, and actions. Our goal is to sustain energy naturally and organically from the moment we open our eyes each morning until we call it a day. Throughout the day, we don't want to overthink and we don't want to think too little. We want to be in a flow state at work, just like the flow states athletes are searching for when they're racing. What's amazing is that flow is always available to us. Learning the proper breathing exercise to get into and stay in flow at the workplace is a tremendous source of personal and professional revenue. Learning how to biohack into flow states before a big meeting or conference call will allow you to make the best choices moment by moment. We can all achieve this level of clarity and inner calm by using our breathing to repattern our parasympathetic nervous system.

Turn on Your Fountain of Youth

The system that slows our heart rate, directs digestion, and conserves energy is the parasympathetic nervous system, sometimes called the rest-and-digest system. When we work with this vital system, we become more dynamic, slow the monkey mind, stall cellular aging, and live a longer, happier life. And the way we train our parasympathetic nervous system is by breathing through the nose and exercising and strengthening the diaphragm muscle.

One way to find out how well our parasympathetic nervous system is doing is to measure our heart-rate variability—the space between heartbeats. The longer the pause between beats, the better our rest and digest system functions. When we slow our breathing and our heart rate, we also expand the transformational spaces between each heartbeat. We do this by properly engaging the diaphragm muscle, which activates the vagus nerve. Working together, this core muscle and cranial nerve create an internal fountain of youth. There's even a ten-year study that showed that deep-breathing practices extended the lives of cancer patients.[2]

Vagus means "wandering" in Latin, and the word fits because this nerve travels from the brain stem, down each side of the neck, across the chest, and into the abdomen. The vagus nerve is an essential part of the parasympathetic system, responsible for calming us down after a fight-or-flight episode. Think of it as our brakes or our air-conditioning system, slowing us down or keeping us cool in heated situations. And it also communicates with all our major organs (you'll learn more about this in Chapter Two). Vagal tone is basically the responsiveness of our vagus nerve, and strong vagal tone means great resilience. This is the science behind the resilience training that's becoming so popular in corporate settings and athletic competitions.

Transformation Starts with Breath

By strengthening our diaphragm, we tone the vagal nerve, improve physical health, heighten cognitive ability, feel better about ourselves, get out of our own way, and fulfill our passion and purpose. We can be the smartest person in the world, but without the emotional intelligence that comes from being calm, centered, and present, we'll be swimming upstream our entire lives. When we combine our knowledge and experience with conscious breathing, we heal, grow, and transform.

$$IQ + EQ = New\ You$$

Full, deep breaths massage our gut, and when our gut is relaxed and happy, we think good thoughts. By breathing

---

Breathing Rates

Averaging more than twelve breaths per minute activates our fight-or-flight system. Since the average person inhales and exhales from fifteen to twenty times a minute, most people are operating in fight-or-flight all day long.

When we're in this hypervigilant state, our body and mind believe we're in danger and we kick into survival mode biochemically and physiologically. The fight-or-flight (sympathetic) system was designed for emergencies, but it's become the dominant operating system for many in our culture. As a result, stress has become the leading cause of chronic and mental illnesses.

20 breaths per minute x 60 = 1,200 × 24 = 28,800
High stress on all levels of your life

15 breaths per minute × 60 = 900 × 24 = 21,600
Average American stress level, not good

10 breaths per minute × 60 = 600 × 24 = 14,400
Insulated from emotional and mental stressors

5 breaths per minute × 60 = 300 × 24 = 7,200
Meditative mind, optimal human awareness

---

through our nostrils, we raise the quality of our questions and ideas and lower the number of thoughts cruising through our brains every second. Our brains take in eleven million bits of information every second, but we're only aware of about forty of those at any given time. When we're calm and present, our thoughts slow down and our emotions can't overpower our intellect. That alone leads to amazing transformations.

Pranayama in Action

After practicing and teaching conscious breathing for more than a decade, I was convinced it was the most powerful transformational tool available to us. But, at that time, the research community wasn't convinced. So when I was asked to work on a research project at Harvard Medical School with Steven Cope, founder and director of the Institute of Extraordinary Living, and Sat Bir Khalsa, one of the leading yoga researchers in the country, I didn't have to think about my answer. It was an immediate "yes." Before this, Cope's institute studied the effects of yoga in many areas, including music, health care, and schools, and Sat Bir Khalsa had studied yoga's effect on singers, performers, and students in an educational setting.

In the study, we monitored a boys' high school crew team, ages seventeen to eighteen, to see how yoga and yoga breathing would affect their performance. The boys practiced the breathing techniques while rowing on indoor machines called ergometers for a distance of two kilometers. By the end of the three-month study, the athletes' 2k erg scores dropped by an average of twenty-two seconds! They'd shaved off more than twice as many seconds as the national average for athletes at their level.

The coach and the athletes were blown away by the rapid improvement, but the boys' parents were blown away by something else. Parents were reporting that their sons were being nicer at home, offering to take the trash out and mow the lawn, and getting along better with their siblings. Their parents loved the change and wanted to know if we were doing something in the study that would cause these mood and behavioral changes. The only things the boys were doing in the study that they hadn't done before were yoga and yoga breathing on the erg. So we got the best of both worlds: the improvement in the sport as well as positive changes in mental and emotional states of being, resulting in the perfect student athlete.

When we use pranayama breathing, we activate the parasympathetic system. In addition to being our rest-and-digest system, it maintains homeostasis, or balance. In pranayama, we must breathe through our nose, which induces creative thoughts and makes us feel calm and comfortable. It also strengthens the muscles we use to inhale and exhale, which takes pressure off our cardiovascular system. When our heart rate and blood pressure are stable, our brain can be present and receive the moment. It's in these moments that we have the ability to re-pattern thoughts and behaviors if we so choose. This is classic neuroplasticity. Our brain has the ability to change continuously throughout our life, and so does our heart. The *way* they change has a lot to do with the way we breathe and the way our autonomic nervous system operates. This system has two branches, the parasympathetic and the sympathetic. Slowly breathing through our nose balances these branches.

When we breathe through our mouth, we experience a mild form of hyperventilation, and when we breathe fast, our brain tells our heart to beat fast, which elevates our blood pressure.

Next, our brain sends all our stored energy to our muscles and bones and slows the process of digestion to compensate for this energy diversion. Our thoughts become unhealthy and fear-based, and we feel agitated, aggressive, or defensive. We're ready to fight or flee.

Mouth breathing is the body's alarm system. It's like hitting the panic button. It activates the stress response that signals the body to release hormones related to fight-or-flight. The chronic use of this system has resulted in an increase in chronic diseases and the earlier onset of diseases. The overuse of these hormones causes elevated inflammation levels, which are at the root of these problems. Not so long ago, people were rarely diagnosed with chronic illness until their mid- to late sixties. Now people are not only being diagnosed with chronic illness in their forties and fifties, but they're also being diagnosed with *multiple* chronic illness conditions.

Building Resilience and Peace of Mind

Professionally, my life with breath has introduced me to a wide variety of industries and performance dynamics, age brackets ranging from nine to eighty-six, and levels of health and fitness ranging from people with chronic illness to elite athletes.

I've noticed that a lot of the CEOs and business owners I coach are athletic and many of them played competitive sports in high school or college. In every case, the same pranayama techniques that I use when I coach elite athletes work for the executives and industry leaders. Using breathing techniques, they learn to reduce stress, build resilience, and improve executive functioning and emotional intelligence. They experience firsthand that breathing through their noses and engaging their diaphragm elevates the quality of their thoughts and decreases the overall number of thoughts rushing through their brains.

This centered mind-set encourages us to ask more and better questions instead of thinking we have all the answers. When we inhale slowly, we stabilize our mental powers of clarity, concentration, and memory. This heightens our executive functioning skills and makes them easily accessible.

The faster we breathe, the more alert our brains are for potential threats and the more fear-based thinking is evoked. In this mind-set, we ignore creative thoughts and potential solutions because our brains are focused on immediate survival. Our heart rate rises, our brain releases adrenaline and our mind spins with thoughts, most of them unhelpful. And it's hard to stop a speeding train. If we continue to strengthen this feedback loop with chronic stress, it can be very difficult to shut off. Over time, the self-regulatory part of the brain becomes damaged, and so does our ability to make good choices. I believe this is the reason we've adopted such poor lifestyle habits with regard to our health and well-being.

Fast, shallow mouth breathing is one of the most efficient ways to wear out your brain, and we're seeing the effects of this as the incidence of mental illnesses and brain disorders rises.[3] We need to take care of the brain and stop all the stressing and overthinking. And we do that by breathing slowly through our noses.

BE'ing YOU Exercise
(Allow twenty minutes)

Practicing this exercise will shift your perceptions. You will not only become aware of new answers to old questions but also tune in to new and deeper questions that will lead to more knowledge of self.

1. Lie on your back on the floor, with your arms and legs in the most comfortable position for you. You may want to place a pillow beneath your knees, but avoid using one for your head unless you have neck issues that require it. Cover yourself with a blanket, close your eyes and relax.

2. Breathe slowly through your nose and release and relax your eyes, cheeks, lips, and jaw. Take ten full breaths.

3. Silently "whisper" the words *soft belly, soft belly, soft belly*, and release and relax the emotional content of the gut with compassion. Take ten full breaths.

4. Breathing as slowly as possible, inhale for a count of three, hold your breath in for a count of three, exhale for a count of three, and hold your breath out for a count of three. Take ten full breaths.

5. Relax into yourself and notice and witness your brain-wave activity. Don't judge, compare, or label. Just sit back in your brain and watch the movie in your head.

6. Hang in there with the experience and keep coming back from sensations or distractions that attempt to slow the process of deep relaxation.

7. If you fall asleep, that's okay, but try to remain "present" and awake in the theta state of being not fully awake nor fully asleep. This is the perfect brainwave for relearning.

8. As you come out of this posture, repeat silently the phrase "I love you" several times to give voice to what's present in your heart.

You Gotta Feel It to Heal It

In my younger years, before I had the great fortune to study yoga and meditation at the Kripalu Center for Yoga and Health, I tried very hard to avoid feeling negative emotions. I'd grown up in a competitive environment, and at some point in my childhood I learned that winning was the end-all and that I had to compete and prove myself to others, always looking for approval. I also learned that winners are brave. So, not only did I stop myself from showing fear, but I also did everything I could to avoid feeling it.

I lived like this for twenty years before I relaxed my brainwave activity enough to *notice* the patterns of fear and powerlessness that permeated my life. Before I attempted to dismantle these patterns, I learned how to breathe, feel, and relax. While practicing yoga and conscious breathing, I also learned new skills for coping with the competitive part of life. After some initial resistance, I began to see that in order to heal and transform, I had to feel my way out. I couldn't think my way out. I had to be willing to ride the waves of emotion, and through pranayama I was able to do that.

At Kripalu, I learned that, fundamentally, the brain works by repeating yesterday today. Every day we have about sixty-thousand thoughts, and many of them are the same day after day. We can repeat the same types of questions and arrive at the same types of answers forever unless we consciously choose to change the pattern. Without making this choice, not much transformation is going to happen.

When I chose to change my old thought patterns, my first new awareness was how powerful nasal breathing is and how important the fundamentals of oxygen and carbon dioxide are to the brain and cardiovascular system. My goal was to slow my brainwave activity without falling asleep. I wanted to consciously take myself from the fast beta waves to the slower alpha waves. Over time, I focused on slowing my brainwaves down to theta, which are the slowest brainwaves we can have prior to being in a state of deep sleep. When we're in a deep sleep, we have the slowest brainwaves, called delta waves.

Controlled breathing and mindful movement are very efficient ways to slow down the brainwaves. In theta brain waves, we're in a state of awareness where we're not fully awake or fully asleep. It's the perfect brainwave activity for reprogramming our brains. It allows us to become our own therapists and heal and transform our perceptions of the world and ourselves.

As I practiced pranayama, the breath held me so that I could explore more and more moments of peace, compassion, authenticity, and higher self expression in safe spaces. And in those spaces, I learned that I'm okay. The breathing practices revealed a weird perfection to all of my perceived imperfections and limiting beliefs. The world became a safe place, and I remembered that I don't have to compete against myself or anyone else if I choose not to play that game.

Neuroplasticity, changing how neurons and synapses are wired, allows us to rewrite our stories. We can replace victimhood with victory. When I shifted my perception from "life is about competition" to "life is about compassion," my whole life changed. In deep states of stress-free relaxation, my neurons rewire my brain to switch off unhealthy competition and turn on healthy compassion.

And it turns out that the secret to a healthy competitive mind state *is* compassion. Transforming ourselves from competitive to compassionate dissolves the patterns of "I'm not good enough, not smart enough, not athletic enough." All negative thought forms are based in competition, and no matter what area of life we're competing in, we're competing against ourselves. It's never about anyone else.

The Incredible Lightness of Breathing

The more we use conscious breathing, the more emotionally balanced we become and the more "lighthearted" we feel. This leads to healthier and happier thoughts and wiser choices. The pranayama techniques work muscles and organs deep inside us, which seems to accelerate the transformational process and invite the brain and heart to work together as a team. As our brain becomes aware of the "light" version of ourselves, it repatterns old thought circuits that are often at the root of unhelpful behaviors like self-sabotage.

Yesterday's events should not stop us from being fully present today. They also shouldn't dictate our future unless we choose that old thought pattern. The cycle of stress and loss of the mind-body connection provides the platform for re-creating negative thoughts, feelings, and behaviors. With breath and balance, we can free ourselves from our biography and become more and more present with what's really going on in each moment. When we're deeply connected with ourselves and living mindfully, we're the witness of old thoughts and behaviors; we're not the enslaved participants. That's when we see the dance of pleasure and pain playing outside of us. That's when we know that everyone in our life is perfectly placed to teach us how to heal our lives and be at peace.

In Chapter Two, we'll look at how breathing affects every organ and system in our bodies.

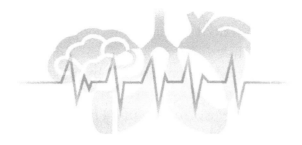

Chapter Two

Our Breathing Determines Our Health and Vitality

"If I had to limit my advice on healthier living to just one tip, it would be simply to learn how to breathe correctly."

— DR. ANDREW WEIL

WHEN WAS THE LAST TIME you woke up feeling great? Has it been a few days? A month? Years? Not many people in the modern world awaken feeling energized and inspired to greet the new day. That's about to change for you.

Over the past fifteen years, I've been at the forefront of the movement to bring yoga breathing into many new arenas, including business and athletics, to improve health and human performance. The body of scientific evidence that mindful breathing provides miraculous benefits is continually expanding. This chapter summarizes a handful of the physical benefits that dramatically improve health and performance.

Breathing is something we rarely think about or talk about because our bodies do it for us. Most people don't think about breathing until they have an illness or disease that makes breathing difficult. My intention is to bring greater awareness to why conscious breathing is critical for optimal health and necessary for peak performance in all areas of our lives. What sets breathing apart from other automatic body functions is that it's the only one we can override and control. Our autonomic nervous system tends to be "sympathetic" dominant, which basically means that it's easily excited. With mindful breathing, we can deliberately shift our nervous systems so that our parasympathetic system is dominant. By doing this, we can use breathing to positively affect asthma, psychological and stress-related disorders, hypertension, the autonomic nervous system, and even our immune function.[4]

Seven Physical Health Benefits from A *Life With Breath*

1. Conserve Energy

Our goal is to conserve energy and avoid wasting it. We all start every morning with a finite amount of energy to use each day. If that energy were in the form of a stack of wood, our goal would be to keep the coals hot and stable and burn as little wood as we need to be at our best. As we age, we have less wood—or energy—to burn. With each log we save, we strengthen our immune system and block the buildup of inflammation. We can support our bodies' natural rhythms and balance with various breathing exercises throughout the day. The body and the brain need to take a break every 90 to 120 minutes. Some of the benefits of taking breaks include greater mental alertness, higher productivity, and deeper, more restful sleep.

2. Reduce Heart Rate and Blood Pressure

When we slow our breathing, we reduce our heart rate and blood pressure, which increases our heart-rate variability. (See Chapter One for a refresher on heart-rate variability.) This allows our calming, cooling parasympathetic nervous system to be dominant, even when we're exercising, negotiating a high-stakes deal, or having an emotionally charged conversation. Keeping our heart rate and blood pressure down can also lower the risk of suffering a stroke or a brain aneurysm.

When we maintain a lower heart rate during the day, we produce less cortisol and adrenaline, our bodies are less acidic, and we have more serotonin and fewer free radicals. That means that at night our brains can do maintenance instead of doing repairs. Day and night, we want to have as much serotonin as we can so that when we *do* get excited and our bodies produce cortisol, we have the right hormonal balance to keep our heart rates down.

In a study conducted on medical students in India, the researchers found that practicing left nostril breathing—one of many pranayama breathing techniques—increases heart rate variability (HRV), improves vagal tone, and promotes cardio-vascular health.[5]

3. Change Gene Expression

Scientists have proved that we can turn genes on and off with the choices we make. Eating anti-inflammatory foods like green leafy vegetables turns on gene processes that prevent heart disease, diabetes, Alzheimer's, and arthritis. Breathing slowly and deeply through the nose is also anti-inflammatory and can change the expression of our genes that influence immune function and the ability to metabolize energy.

The science of epigenetics, which studies the interaction between our environment and our genes, has found that *from 70 percent to 90 percent of all chronic disease is being caused by our lifestyle and environment.* Where we live, how and what we eat, drink, and breathe, and what we do and think all determine our health. No one gets sick by chance. Everything we do has an effect on our health.

A study conducted by a team of scientists in Norway found that certain pranayama breathing techniques create "rapid and significant changes" in gene expression in peripheral blood lymphocytes (PBMCs) when study participants practiced specific breathing techniques and related practices.[6]

The latest research shows that physiological mechanisms like oxidative stress, inflammation, and mitochondrial dysfunction are at the root of all diseases. When we breathe slowly and deeply, through our noses, we put out the fire that causes oxidative stress and inflammation. Deep, slow breathing also feeds and detoxes the mitochondria, tiny organelles in most of our cells that handle the biochemical processes of respiration and energy production.

4. Strengthen the Immune System

Practically every month I see a new research study that shows that yoga, pranayama, or meditation have a positive influence on our immune systems. For example, researchers in the Netherlands found that the sympathetic nervous system and the immune system could be influenced with breathing techniques, meditation, and exposure to cold temperatures. As reported in Proceedings of the National Academy of Sciences of the United States of America (PNAS):

> Healthy volunteers practicing the learned techniques exhibited profound increases in the release of

epinephrine which, in turn, led to increased production of anti-inflammatory mediators and subsequent dampening of the proinflammatory cytokine response elicited by intravenous administration of bacterial endotoxin.

The research team concluded, "This study could have important implications for the treatment of a variety of conditions associated with excessive or persistent inflammation, especially autoimmune diseases in which therapies that antagonize pro-inflammatory cytokines have shown great benefit."[7]

5. Slow the Aging Process

We're not making as many cells today as we did yesterday, so we want to stall the aging process wherever we can. The faster we breathe, the more heat we create, and that heat burns cells and dries out bones. The slower we breathe, the less energy we burn and the more slowly we age.[8]

Breathing through the nose amplifies the amazing power of the vagus nerve. Toning this nerve stalls the aging process in all the cells in your body and your brain. Increasing the tone of your vagus nerve is one of the most important actions you can take to perform at the highest level possible with the least amount of stress on your body and mind.

6. Burn Fat

When we're breathing slowly and deeply through our noses, our brains relax and tell our bodies to burn fat instead of sugar. As we move through our daily routine, it's important to be in fat-burning mode so we don't run out of energy before the end of the day. When we get up each morning, we have about thirty minutes of potential energy in the form of sugars and about thirty days of energy stored in fat. When our breathing rates are constantly signaling the brain for a sympathetic response, our body will burn sugar instead of fat, depleting our energy. In search of more energy, we turn to energy substitutes like sugar and caffeine, which have myriad negative consequences, including disrupting our sleep.

While conducting a study to determine what happens to fat when we lose it, researchers at the University of New South Wales found that our lungs are our main excretory organ for fat. We lose the weight on our exhale. And based on everything I'm revealing in this book, a nasal exhale is more efficient and effective than a mouth exhale. They concluded, "Losing weight requires unlocking the carbon stored in fat cells, thus reinforcing that often heard refrain of 'eat less, move more.'"[9] I have seen firsthand that even for people who can't exercise, the breathing practices alone can accelerate their weight loss.

7. Sleep Deeply

The negative effects of sleep deprivation on health and performance are well-documented, but many Americans are sleep-deprived more often than not. Changing our breathing can dramatically improve our sleep.

When we stimulate the vagus nerve with deep breathing and do gentle neck rolls, we tell our brains to secrete the hormone serotonin. We need to have a high level of cooling serotonin during the day to fall asleep and sleep through the night. When we're not sleeping well, it's often because our levels of cortisol and adrenaline are high, and that causes our systems to overheat.

A study conducted by the Department of Psychobiology and Methodology at the University of Malaga showed that yoga practice improves sleep quality and modulates cortisol levels.[10] In another study, conducted by Harvard Medical School's Division of Sleep Medicine, people with chronic insomnia were studied to see if a daily yoga practice would help them to sleep. After practicing the yoga and breathing techniques for eight weeks, the participants showed significant improvements in sleep efficiency and total sleep time. They also awoke fewer times during the night and stayed awake for shorter periods before falling back to sleep.[11]

Reap the Rewards by Developing Your Biggest Muscle

Our diaphragm, the largest muscle in our body, is located below the lungs and heart and above the liver, gallbladder, stomach, and spleen. When we take shallow breaths or breathe through our mouths, we don't engage the diaphragm and it doesn't move. When we breathe deeply through our noses, our diaphragm pushes down, and with each inhalation, it massages our gastrointestinal tract and stimulates strong digestive flow so our bodies can remove mucus, phlegm, fat, and inflammation from the inner walls of our organs.

In addition to playing a vital role in breathing, developing the diaphragm muscle gives us tremendous lower back support and helps to keep our spines straight, which take the strain off the muscles in our trunk, abdomen, hips, and buttocks.[12]

As our diaphragm muscle gets stronger, our rib cage becomes more elastic, and that allows our lungs to expand and take in an enormous amount of oxygen. Most people are taking in only a small fraction of the five quarts of oxygen that our lungs can hold. The combination of a super-strong diaphragm muscle and an elastic rib cage adds up to a boatload of energy and vitality.

So learning how to train that diaphragm muscle on the inhale to really push down and holding your breath in for a few seconds are going to expand and reshape your rib cage so you can reduce the number of breaths you take every minute. The latest science recommends you aim for twelve breaths per minute, but you can do better. Make your first goal to get to twelve, and then focus on dropping that number down to four slow, deep breaths a minute. The breathing techniques in Chapter Three and the daily practices in the thirty-day program will allow this to happen naturally.

Oxygen is one of nature's miracle drugs, and when our diaphragm is strong, we can move oxygen deeper into our muscles, tissues, and nervous system, which provides us with enormous power.

The diaphragm is also the main muscle that connects our upper and lower body. The stronger this muscle becomes, the greater connection we have to the parts of our body below the navel. Our diaphragm is also our strongest core muscle, so when it's strong, we can conserve the energy we'd otherwise need to contract all our other core muscles. A strong diaphragm also gives us a broad range of motion in our lower backs, hips, and buttocks, while contracting the other core muscles constricts our range of motion.

Small Changes Make Big Differences

Pranayama breathing changes our biology and our psychology. It literally changes our story and the way we see and interact with the people around us. One of the most dramatic examples I've seen of pranayama in action is how a company of more than nine hundred employees was transformed by fifty leaders who I was working with one-on-one, using conscious breathing practices.

When I started working with this company, the Wednesday-afternoon meetings were all about defending turf and attacking anyone who threatened to touch "your" piece of the pie. The meetings were characterized by personal insults and even bullying and shaming. Keep in mind that these were the company's "successful" leaders.

About three months after I started teaching fifty company leaders my breathing practices, mindful foundational movement, and deep relaxation skill sets, one of the owners called me into his office. He said that the way people were interacting at the Wednesday meetings with staff leadership had become much more positive and productive even though he hadn't done anything differently that he was aware of. "I can almost see some of them wanting to blurt something out, but then it's like they catch themselves and take a deep breath before they say something," he said. "And instead of competing to be right, they're cooperating."

He said that the meetings had more human connection, more eye contact, and that the people even had better posture, sitting up instead of sinking into their chairs. "The energy of the meetings has changed so much that people stick around afterward and talk about their kids and what they have planned for the weekend," he said.

And there was one other benefit the owners never expected to realize from this new way of breathing, thinking, and leading was bringing to the company. In a down economy, when other companies were letting people go or closing their doors, this company became the most successful in its field.

Reaching New Heights

The breath can be used as a tool to keep us tethered to Earth and the cycles of nature that unfold every twenty-four hours. Our bodies are naturally in cycle with the rising of the sun, the setting of the moon, and what happens in between. Our bodies are going through a biochemical and physiological process throughout the day that's rooted in our circadian and ultradian rhythms. As the sun rises, we move into a fire or heating energy. There's a midmorning energy, midday energy, midafternoon energy, early-evening energy and, finally, a cooling energy when the moon is high.

As the sun and moon dance across our sky, we can apply different breath techniques to keep our energy and awareness attuned to Mother Nature, the most powerful force on the planet. Tuning in to these organic flows of energy enliven the mind-body in a relaxed way.

In the morning hours when the sun is rising in the sky and the moon's energy is turned down, our body is heating up with the sun. Our energy levels are high. It's a great time to exercise, and most of us work more efficiently in the morning. At this time of day, we work on our exhalations to stay cool and conserve energy that we'll need in the afternoon.

In the afternoon, the sun is descending and the rising moon has a cooling effect on the body. We begin to experience a lag in mental capacity and feel like we need a nap. At this point, we can do breathing techniques that create heat, more fire to counteract the flow of the day.

When staying connected to nature, the mind-body is more in sync with our heart's powerful, supporting, fearless messages to grow beyond yesterday's thoughts today.

Beginning now, while you're reading, consciously increase the length of your inhalations and try to double the length of your exhalations, training yourself to take fewer breaths per minute. Pay attention to how full you can make your lungs with each inhale and how empty you can make them with each exhale. By doing this, you're alkalizing your blood and removing as much acidity as you can. This scrubs your blood of impurities. I'm convinced that conscious breathing is what's kept me from getting sick for the past twenty years.

Making it a habit to breathe through your nose and slow your breathing will have a profound impact on your health and on your life. You can begin both these practices immediately. Whenever you realize you're breathing through your mouth, switch over to nostril breathing and take a moment or two to consciously slow the rate of your breathing and deepen the inhalations and exhalations. The beauty of this is that it becomes a part of everything you do. While at rest, while at play, while exercising, while working, consciously change your breath and watch your physical, mental, and emotional health transform. This is life with breath.

In Chapter Three, you'll learn more about the breathing mechanics for great mental and physical health and peak performance in your daily life and work.

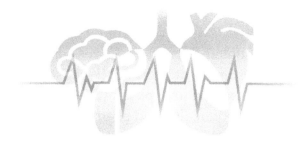

Chapter Three

The Mechanics of Conscious Breathing

"The most expensive bed is a hospital bed"
— STEVE JOBS

WHAT WE CALL LIFE begins with our first inhalation and ends with our last exhalation. These two breaths are the bookends to our story of life. And when you get farther down this path, you'll discover that our story is really all we have. How we interact with the breaths in between will determine the quality of our lives.

For most people, breathing is a shallow, superficial process; they use only the upper portion of the lungs instead of filling them to the full capacity, which is five quarts. Most adults fill only a small fraction of their lungs, and that's one of the reasons so many people suffer from fatigue, foggy thinking, and unhealthy choices.

Although we breathed deeply when we were babies, poor breathing patterns develop over time because of sedentary lifestyles, accumulated tension and stress, and lack of attention to the present moment. This shallow breathing deprives the body of both oxygen and prana (life-force energy), leading to deterioration of health and premature aging. The good news is that by practicing conscious breathing methods, we can retrain ourselves so that deep, slow breathing becomes natural to us again.

Breathing is the most undervalued tool used for physical and mental health. How we breathe dictates the physiologic response from several key systems in our bodies.

Breathe through Your Nose

When we were born, we all breathed diaphragmatically through our noses. Watch infants or young children breathe—they breathe with their belly. Now watch adults—they breathe with their mouth or the upper portion of their lungs, rarely engaging the lower portion of the abdomen in the process. Every animal on Earth breathes through its nose for its entire life unless it's hunting, being hunted, or sick. But, in our culture, most adolescents and adults breathe through their mouths.

Somewhere along the line, people lost the mind-body connection yielded through breathing. That's why we get lost in our heads with thoughts, feelings, and emotions that become the drivers of choices resulting in unhealthy lifestyles. The most self-aware and spiritually aware people breathe through their noses. They are visibly calm, centered, and relaxed. They practice self-care and self-regulation. And it all begins by setting the moment in motion by inhaling and exhaling through our nostrils.

When I'm working with clients, whether they're athletes, executives, or celebrities, I incorporate nostril-breathing exercises to help them maintain the mind-body connection and create balance within the autonomic nervous system. This, in turn, keeps the brain tuned to the subtle energy flow of the planet. We begin to experience more energy, but it's calm energy, whereas breathing through the mouth tells the brain to prepare for battle or run for our lives.

Another way that breathing through our nose and mouth creates different physiological effects is that only nasal belly breathing moves the abdominal diaphragm downward when we inhale, literally massaging the gut 20,500 times a day. The psoas muscle runs through our gut, connecting the upper and lower halves of our body. Physically, it's responsible for good posture and stability. Mentally and emotionally, it's connected to fear and anxiety. Just as our belly is known as "the seat of our soul," this muscle is known as "the muscle of our soul." Emotions are stored in our gut, and proper diaphragmatic breathing massages the organs and muscles associated with this region, keeping them supple, flexible, and open to the present moment.

Like all movements in the body, the mechanics of our inhale involve a muscular contraction. Every inhalation begins with a contraction of our external intercostal muscle and our diaphragm. This allows our rib cage to lift and our diaphragm to drop into our abdomen. Practice attempting to access the lower lobes of the lungs before drawing the breath up toward the pit of your throat. This breathing technique is designed to maximize certain structural effects of inhaling and exhaling.

The quality of the exhale involves our ability to contract primarily our rectus abdominals, which are paired muscles running vertically on each side of the abdomen. It's the area where we try to have "six-pack abs." The exhale removes toxic wastes and stabilizes your mind's activity.

Length, Depth and Pace Matter

How we breathe factors into how well we oxygenate our cells, whether we're burning fat or sugar, the release of hormones, heart rates, lactic acid buildup, cardiovascular and digestive function, and so much more. When we're breathing through our nose, we're also activating our vagus nerve, which releases serotonin to support rest-and-digest functions. It's very cooling, so it keeps the heat of our exercise or exertion at a moderate level. In most exercise sessions or high-stress situations, the heating, sympathetic response is overstimulated, and that hinders digestion.

To take full advantage of the health and power our breathing can produce, we want to pay attention to three primary factors: the length, depth, and pace of our breath. These three variables set the tone for our autonomic nervous system.

1. Length
The length of our breath is a reflection of the types of thoughts moving across our brow.

2. Depth
The depth of our breath regulates the exchange of oxygen and carbon dioxide.

3. Pace
The pace of our breath signals sympathetic or parasympathetic activity.

The Length of Your Inhale and Exhale

The longer we inhale, the greater vitality we have. Our heart rate will remain low and our digestive fire will be free from mucus, phlegm, fat, and other impediments that rob us of the energy we need to move our bodies and fully engage our minds. Lengthening the inhale by slowing it down also stimulates the parasympathetic nervous system, which is calming. But we get these benefits only when we breathe through our nose. We also have to inhale through our nose for our brain to make an anti-inflammatory substance called nitric oxide that dilates our bronchial tubes, making it easier to take in more oxygen.

The longer we exhale, the more serotonin we create. Exhaling slowly also gives our body a chance to absorb the oxygen molecule that's in the carbon dioxide we're exhaling. After we complete an exhalation, if we hold our breath for a few seconds before inhaling, our brain will search for oxygen in our lungs' alveoli sacs and in the tissue of our organs and muscles. What's beautiful about this is that while we hold out the exhale, our brain is incinerating stale air that hasn't been fully exchanged. And when our brain uses that stale air as fuel, it opens up that space for our next inhalation to penetrate it with the fresh oxygen our cells need.

The Depth of Your Inhale

In addition to slowing down our inhale and exhale, we want to inhale as fully as we can. Shallow breathing not only deprives us of the energy that oxygen provides, but it also leads to a weak diaphragm muscle. This is of major importance because our diaphragm muscle affects the quality of movement for six hundred muscles and 206 bones.

We can get an amazing cardio workout just by inhaling through our nose for as long as we can. When our lungs feel full, we tell our nose to inhale a little more—and then a little more—and feel our lungs expand. There are microscopic openings at the top of the lungs that are constantly burning carbon dioxide, so there's always a little space being made for more oxygen. You'll feel some pressure and it will be challenging, but the more you practice this breathing, the easier it will be, and the payoffs are huge.

When you begin this practice, you may not be able to sustain it for too long, but even a few tiny inhales will exercise and strengthen the muscles that allow you to fully expand your lungs. These muscles will develop with training just like all your other muscles. When you stop the inhalation and return to your regular breathing, you'll notice that your airflow is unobstructed and you feel calm, energized, and focused.

The Pace of Your Breathing

Every breath we take tells our brain something about our emotional state. The hypothalamus gland in our brain is vigilantly monitoring the pace of our breath. When we're breathing slowly and deeply, it lets our brain know we're safe, and that keeps cortisol levels low and generates a sense of ease in all the systems of our body. So the pace of our breath is extremely important.

The fewer breaths we take each minute and the more efficiently our body utilizes oxygen and carbon dioxide, the better we'll perform in all life's arenas. For endurance athletes, aka humans, the one nutrient that's critical to our overall performance is oxygen. But we also need carbon dioxide for our body to function properly. For our body to maintain the right balance of oxygen and carbon dioxide, we have to breathe through our nose. And remember that breathing through our nose also creates nitric acid, which lowers our blood pressure and dramatically increases our lungs' ability to absorb oxygen.[13]

The faster we breathe, the more often our heart beats. The slower we breathe, the less often our heart beats. When our heart beats fast, our brain senses danger, and this perpetuates the chronic state of fight-or-flight that many people experience when there's no real threat of danger. On the other hand, when we breathe slowly, we lower our heart rate, and that tells our brain to relax, expand awareness, and learn new things.

The length, depth, and pace of each breath affect every aspect of your health and have a dynamic effect on how you perform in all areas of your life. By consciously controlling your breathing, over time you'll train and repattern your nervous system so that deep, slow breathing becomes your norm.

Training for Life, Love, Work, and Sports

Thousands of years ago, yogis learned that to raise energy levels in the body, they needed to skillfully manipulate the breathing process. Breathing exercises (pranayama) were developed and practiced to allow the mind to become sensitive to where the energy is strongest in the body at any given moment. Yoga scientists discovered that "energy follows awareness." Leading psychiatrists in the West have scientifically proved this profound statement.

After teaching the CEOs and athletes to train their respiratory system first, they began seeing improvements in their health, including brain function and cardiovascular, respiratory, and digestive health. Stress and its debilitating effects on the mind are something that business leaders need to address, and 30-Day

Breath as Medicine program is the perfect prescription with no negative side effects.

The most beneficial way to improve our health and performance is to train our respiratory system. As this system becomes more dynamic on inhale and exhale, our cardiovascular system won't have to work so hard, so our heart rate doesn't rise as high, and when it does go up, it resets back down very quickly.

The Most Effective and Efficient Physical Training Order

1. Respiratory

2. Cardiovascular

3. Muscular

4. Skeletal

Training Your Respiratory System

Slow down, let your ego dissolve, and work at the pace that's correct for your current cardiovascular condition. If you have to open your mouth to get enough air, you're pushing too hard. If you're panting, you're doing more harm than good in the long run, both literally and metaphorically. Instead, put your focus and commitment on developing your diaphragm muscle. You'll live a heck of a lot longer, and you'll probably bypass a lot of the depression, the Alzheimer's, the dementia, the schizophrenia, and the other brain diseases that are on the rise among the older population.

As your diaphragm muscle gets stronger, your rib cage is going to become more elastic and that will allow your lungs to expand and take in an enormous amount of oxygen. The combination of a superstrong diaphragm muscle and an elastic rib cage adds up to a boatload of energy and vitality.

Training the diaphragm muscle on the inhale to really push down and holding your breath in for a few seconds is going to expand and reshape your rib cage so you can reduce the number of breaths you take each minute. The latest science suggests you aim for twelve breaths per minute, but you can do better. Make your first goal to get to twelve and then focus on dropping that number down to four slow, deep breaths a minute. Doing the 30-day program in Part Two will allow this to happen organically.

In Western culture, training traditionally starts with muscular and skeletal systems, instead of the respiratory and cardio systems, and that creates heat. As your heart detects the rising cortisol and acidity, it starts to beat faster to bring in more oxygen and cool the fire. And your respiratory muscles are going to have to work harder.

But when you train your respiratory system first by using breathing techniques and strategies, your heart rate will be lower during intense activity, and when your heart rate is lower, your blood pressure will rise less during intense activity, which means your body will have more alkalinity and less acidity, which allows your cells to live longer. Keeping your heart rate low also allows you to learn. When your heart rate is high and adrenaline is present in the brain, there's very little learning taking place. And, ideally, you want to learn something new or gain some new awareness every time you work out.

When you train the respiratory system first and the cardiovascular system second, you don't wear out your moving parts and you don't overincinerate muscle mass, which shortens the life of your cells.

Since we're talking about "life with breath," we even want to focus on breathing during exercise. We're going to work on transitioning you from mouth breathing during exercise to nasal breathing during exercise. The foundational practice here is breathing diaphragmatically as described earlier in this chapter. Here's how you bring breath into your exercise routines.

Training Sequence

1. Warm Up with Breath: Warm-ups play a vital role in preparing your body for the workout.

2. Train with Breath: Use nasal breathing to balance the autonomic nervous system and biohack into flow states.

3. Recover with Breath: Integration periods at the end of a workout are key for preparing your body for your next workout.

Hacking into Flow

You can hack your way into flow, expand space and time, and silence the inner critic that exists in your left prefrontal cortex. The way you do this is by using certain breathing techniques that create the five chemicals that interact to create flow.[14] Whenever these five chemicals come together, we're in the zone.

Five Flow Chemicals

1. Serotonin relaxes and creates community in our thought forms.

2. Dopamine is our source of motivation and desire.

3. Endorphins are nature's natural painkiller.

4. Anandamide is called the "bliss molecule."

5. Norepinephrine cuts down all the noise and distraction of what's not important now.

Strategically using conscious breathing techniques primes your body to biohack into a state of flow. Engaging your diaphragm muscle and activating your vagus nerve by breathing through your nose creates the blend of calming serotonin and feel-good dopamine that you need for flow and heart-rate variability.[15] When you're both aroused and relaxed, you're invincible. Athletes, artists, CEOs, engineers and people from every walk of life do amazing things when they're in the flow.

Grounding Techniques

Breathe

1. Watch breathing process closely and clearly. Keep connecting with the different qualities of each breath.

2. Always look to lengthen volume of exchange.

3. Bring inhale to left side of the brain, exhale right side of the belly when breathing process is laboring.

4. Bring inhale to right side of the brain, exhale left side of the belly when you reach your desired intensity.

Relax

1. Inhale slowly to relax and calm the mind.

2. Exhale slowly and relax the body.

3. Relax the major muscles and bones first, and then scan internal landscape from the inside out.

4. Silently repeat the word *relax* to yourself over and over.

Feel

1. Use your mind and body to "feel into" the movement you're about to make before gracefully moving your body from the inside out.

2. Scan your body and feel tension building, and then remove it with your breath or change the angle of power.

3. Feel energy disguised as emotions in each moment. Emotion is the fuel of thoughts.

4. Always feel where your energy is the strongest in any moment and access it through breath, imagery, and visualizing.

Watch

1. Always witness what's happening with compassion for yourself in the present moment.

2. Observe each moment unfolding without the mind's input from the past or future.

3. Watch the mind's tricks; don't let it separate you from the present.

4. Watch the breath and the body before your thoughts and feelings.

Allow

1. Focus only on the present and allow it to unfold.

2. Don't try to understand what's happening energetically.

3. Allow your breath to do more for you as energy levels inevitably drop.

4. Allow yourself to transcend the contractions of electronic created time.

Breathing Practice

Sit on the edge of a firm chair so that your spine is erect.

Roll your shoulder blades up, back, and down several times and begin to let the day go. Let go of any tension in your neck and throat. Gently tilt your head from right to left and back again a few times. Now drop your chin to your chest and then raise it to point upward; repeat this a few times.

Let your eyes close. Focus your attention on your inhale and exhale and consciously slow them down.

As you inhale, feel your diaphragm pressing down and supporting your spine.

Continue to inhale and exhale as slowly as you can. If your head wants to move, let it move. Keep giving your attention to your inhale, feeling it massage and clean your digestive organs.

Now begin to work on your exhale, your ability to let go. Remember that there's one oxygen molecule in the carbon dioxide, so when you exhale slowly through your nose, your brain will extract that oxygen molecule and add it to the two oxygen molecules you get on the inhale, and you'll be aroused and also relaxed.

After the next inhale is complete, hold the breath in for two seconds and alert your mind that you're the CEO and you have the ability to change any behavior that's causing you to age.

When your next exhale is complete, hold the breath out for two seconds. This will incinerate the stale air, detoxing your lungs, organs, and tissues.

On the next inhale, feel the fresh oxygen filling your lungs, and imagine you can see it permeating every cell of your body.

As you inhale, see the best in yourself.

As you exhale, let your image of yourself drop away.

Inhale, hold two seconds

Exhale, hold two seconds.

Do one more round of inhale and exhale.

Let the next breath fill your heart. Because you're probably doing a thousand times better than you give yourself credit for.

This is a great exercise to do while sitting or walking or as a warm-up routine for a more physical form of exercise. It's also a great way to fall asleep at night.

In Part Two, you'll be guided step-by-step through the 30-Day Breath as Medicine program.

My Message To You As You Discover Your "Life With Breath"

Without love, nothing is worth our energy of doing

With love, all is within our being

The mind is focused only on our accomplishments

The heart sees thru all our worldly accomplishments
as trivial games of the ego mind

Life is taking place in an invisible field of pure potential

The potential sits quiet, waiting for us to become as quiet

In that quiet, we remember

We remember something hidden from
us, in us, at our human birth

In the remembering, we forget all judgment
and competitive mind games

We remember we are all one

All one in the same playing the same games

The game is trust. The more we trust, the
more open and fearless life becomes

Our birth . . . our death, simply games of the flesh

Life is about trusting what our 5 senses
bring to each moment, then going into the
field of breath to watch and allow

In the watching, we notice truths and nontruths equally

That balance removes all of our unbalanced
thought forms and emotional debris

Breathe . . . Trust . . . Remember

Breath . . . Trust . . . Remember

The whole universal field is waiting to
reveal itself to you and me

Let's Go Now

Go BE Great!

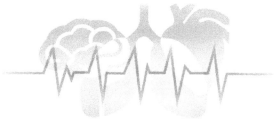

Part Two

The 30-Day Breath-as-Medicine Program

I'VE PROVIDED YOU WITH a series of daily self-care practices for the next thirty days. These practices are designed to deepen your relationship with your breath, begin the process of reestablishing autonomic balance, and provide you with the opportunity to become more self-aware and transform the thoughts, emotions, and behavior that influence your ability to be the best version of yourself.

In this plan, a combination of education and experiential exercises will help you embody the wisdom found through *life with breath*. In addition to the breathing exercises, I've included daily intentions for our physical, mental, emotional, and spiritual selves. These are the P I E S within each section that can help bring awareness to our body, our thoughts, our feelings, and our connection to a greater source. Use these intentions within your daily practice to observe, feel, and transform wherever there is an opportunity for healing and growth.

Every day there will be a new awareness. It won't be easy, yet it's really quite simple. It's hard, but easy enough for anyone to accomplish. Go slow at first and get your legs underneath the information. Practice daily until it becomes part of who you are. Then bring the techniques into every facet of your life. The good, the not so good, the ugly. Let the breath do the work; not you. You just have to learn and practice these techniques to get into a daily routine. Once the brain sees that what you're offering can be trusted, it will look for more ways to integrate these skills into every interpersonal and outerpersonal perception you have about yourself and others. You will start to feel lighter, more lighthearted, but tough in many ways without the need to be negative. You will become grateful for your life on every level, conscious, subconscious, and unconscious. It's all one big adventure. In life with breath, the wind is at your back, gently nudging you forward into fearless adventures. Everything works itself out in our lives, if we can live long enough for the knots to untie themselves.

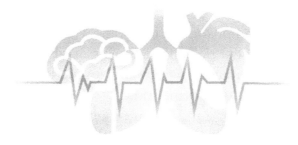

Day 1

*"Why do you stay in prison when
the door is so wide open?"*

— RUMI

EVERY DAY, EVEN EVERY moment if we wish, we have the opportunity to heal and transform ourselves. This journey begins with strong physical and mental posture. Mind-body posture is everything when life is taking us out of balance. From the surface to the deeper levels of the mind-body, holding our balance longer today than yesterday as events unfold is a huge accomplishment. Posture helps us stay clam, use less energy, avoid getting worked up, and ride the waves of discomfort that attempt to temporarily turn us into something we're not. When life starts to shrink us, great spinal posture holds us upright and open, rather than shrinking and closing to the present moment's lesson.

Good physical posture comes from cultivating a long, erect spine, creating more space for breath from our belly to our collarbone. We want to be conscious of our posture, perform good nasal breathing and pay attention to how we're moving the abdominal diaphragm.

As we become more conscious of the anatomy or our breath and the length and posture of our spine, we increase our capacity to take in nutrient-rich air, delivering an abundant supply of oxygen to our brain and thereby improving the mind's ability to focus and process information.

Evolving as we age and mature should be a natural process. Unfortunately, stress and fear start to slip into our thoughts and feelings as we experience the challenges that life brings, and this leads to disease in the body and imbalance in the mind. If we constantly stimulate our stress physiology, we stay in a biochemical state that's meant for emergencies only.

To stall the cellular aging (degeneration) process of the body and brain caused by today's stressors, we first correct our breathing from high and shallow to slow and deep. As the nervous system begins receiving rich levels of oxygen, we begin to restore the balance in body and mind. As the nervous system is repaired and balanced, we can begin to make the shift from a constant state of stress (fight-or-flight), which is our sympathetic nervous system physiology, to a state of calm (heal-and-repair), which is our parasympathetic physiology.

Our beliefs create our biology and our emotional reactions and responses. To remain present and reflective requires intense focus. This includes paying deeper attention to things crossing your mind as they manifest and staying fully in the present moment without longing for the past or dreaming of the future. These are acquired skills that take time and practice. The definition of peace is to accept all that is, exactly as it is, in each moment. The skill lies in not getting caught up in the stories that begin with "if only," or "should've, could've, would've." Instead, accept what is and create a plan for change if needed in the present moment. Be patient, but don't let yourself off the hook too easily. You must be accountable at the deepest levels of yourself.

Fear and resistance are powerful opportunities for growth if you consciously choose to stay with these emotions longer, allowing them the time to deliver their message, to acknowledge what part of yourself is in conflict with your choices. Every answer to every question raised in life is within you; you are immensely more knowledgeable than you give yourself credit for. Look how far you've come!

Invite your full range of emotions. Choose to remain open to perceiving everything as an opportunity for awareness and, in turn, growth. Don't take yourself quite so seriously. Be light. Be lovely. Be in beginner's mind. Be the breath.

Today's Practice

With compassion, remind yourself to breathe as slowly as possible through your nostrils as you go about your day. Become aware of your breathing pattern. What are the length, depth, and pace? Do you know when you're barely breathing? Just watch the breath, and the thoughts that arise moment by moment. Relax and feel the energy of your breath creating, sustaining, and leading you to the next awareness. Sit back in your mind and just observe, without the need to judge your level of expertise or to understand more right now. *Just breathe.*

Your goals are to become conscious of your breath as often as possible throughout the day and to shift from shallow or mouth breathing to breathing through your nose diaphragmatically. When you were a baby, you naturally breathed in this fashion. We go back to our birth with the breath. Begin to develop a relationship with nasal breathing in your daily routines, including exercise, work, play, and rest. Allow your meditative mind to reflect on the vibrational messages of this book. As you rewire your brain and the various systems of the body, you will heal and transform, revealing the new you.

P Tap into a deeper level of awareness and notice the difference between a proper breathing process and an improper one.

I Watch the rise and fall of your thoughts as you slowly deepen your breath.

E Notice the quality of your sensations and feelings when your belly expands and contracts, before your ribs move.

S Relax into yourself, your likes and dislikes, and know they are all teachers in disguise.

Today's Practice Notes

_____

_____

_____

_____

Day 2

"Our inhale is everything! Use the inhale to create the space you require to move through the steps of your life with good posture, your feet on the ground, and an open mind. The open mind sets in motion a new perception of old mental patterns that no longer serve us in healthy ways. As the inhale opens the mind, so go our hearts."

— ED HARROLD

EACH BREATH WE TAKE has a beginning (birth), a middle (life) and an ending (death). Every breath is the completion of one cycle of life. In a twenty-four-hour period, the average person takes 21,600 breaths and has between 50,000 and 80,000 thoughts. The more stressed your mind and body are, the more breaths you take per minute and the faster you age. Slow the breath and relax the mind and body.

The natural organic expanse between inhale and exhale is a powerful space. Most people are so stimulated that they're not even aware that they have a constant stream of opportunities for transformation in that space. That silence and stillness holds a moment of deep peace. Listen deeply into that space. I like to hold that space open, not placing any thought or feeling there, just simply listening to and feeling the natural fusion of personal power with the unifying creative force of the universe.

Courageously explore this magical space, my friends. This is the place to allow yourself to evolve into self-mastery of anything or everything you're attempting to achieve at this point of your life. It doesn't cost you anything, and it's accessible all the time. Whether you're driving, exercising, working, or playing, this magical space contains messages from your higher self. It contains our hearts' intelligence, but most people don't hear it. To learn to be present and pay attention to the universal space between your inhale and exhale is the beginning of a meditation practice.

We've all heard about the benefits of meditation. It's a gift to you from the Universe. So get started *now*.

✳ *Today's Practice*

Today, we're going to work on improving our inhale. It should be slow and deliberate, not rushed. Imagine you're filling a vase with water. As you fill the vase, the water starts at the bottom and gradually makes its way to the top. Let's think of our inhale in the same way.

Begin inhaling through your nose down into your abdomen. Next, move the diaphragm muscle downward toward the internal abdominal organs, letting the belly swell outward as if you were doing a reverse sit-up. Then on the second half of the inhale, try to expand your rib cage like gills on a fish. Finish the inhale by expanding the upper portion of the lungs just under your collarbone.

Always try to inhale as slowly as possible in the learning stage. Try to inhale slower and slower and notice the details of the process we call inhale. Sit back in your mind's eye and ear and make little notes for yourself on the physical and mental level of what we call inhale.

The goal is to inhale the breath into all three chambers of your torso slowly and deliberately. Repeat for several rounds. Incorporate this practice into your day.

P   Slow everything down and become aware of the muscles you use to inhale and the muscles you use to exhale.

I   Stopping your breath stops your mind. Your mind will sit for you and listen instead of talking.

E   Allow yourself to feel the moment first and apply a meaning or thought second.

S   When you stop your breathing, merge with that quiet space.

Today's Practice Notes

_____

_____

_____

_____

Day 3

*"If you love life, don't waste time, for
time is what life is made up of."*

— BRUCE LEE

KNOW THIS: YOU WERE not born to be average. Your best days are in front of you. Mother Nature removes excess throughout daily, weekly, and monthly cycles as we move around the wheel of the year. Everything that's alive today is needed tomorrow to maintain balance. This universal balance is beyond the perception of our five bodily senses. It happens whether we're aware of it or not, whether we believe in it or not.

We don't have a predetermined destiny. As scientists break information down into smaller and smaller particles, they observe something amazing. The behavior of the tiniest particles is unpredictable. Nobody can predict what will happen next. So don't rule anything out. We're kind of winging this thing called life, so we'll always have some uncertainty, but that's what gives us the ability to mindfully and willfully create the life we desire.

We all wish we had more information about what has come to pass in our lives and why. And we all wish we had more insight into the future. What's important to remember is that we *do* have intuition and the ability to trust our gut and go with the soft whispers of our heart. We can stop listening to the rhetoric of belief systems that no longer serve us and move toward radical self-acceptance, expansion, and healing. It's natural to want a safe future, free of suffering, but pain will always be with us. It's part of being human. So why not learn to perceive pain as a compassionate teacher? Anger will also be with us, so why not make it a tool for working toward peace in our hearts?

Trust that the universe knows what's best for you and surrender the part of yourself that resists this timeless teaching. If you don't have the answers today, it doesn't mean you won't have them tomorrow. Trust, be patient, and accept and love your life as it is today.

✳ *Today's Practice*

Today we're working on the details of the exhale. If you're under higher levels of stress than you're used to, the exhale is the first self-care tool to reset autonomic function. We must start today to slowly lengthen the amount of time it takes to deflate the lungs fully. Yesterday we practiced slowing down the inhale, so today let's practice slowing down the exhale. Be aware that the exhale occurs with the help of all your sit-up muscles. Try to slowly deflate the lungs to completion. Practice completely exhaling only through your nose, then inhaling as slowly as possible. Empty the lungs to completion without strain as many times as you can today.

Try to exhale as slowly as possible and notice the physical and mental sensations that arise. Any time we're learning something new, we go slowly at first. This is no different. The slower the exhale, the less energy we'll need on the next inhale. The first goal is to not have to exhale through the mouth unless it's an emergency situation.

> **P** Slow everything down and focus on the muscles of exhale. Feel these muscles pushing stale energy up and out of the mind-body container.

> **I** Exhale slowly, letting go of the last moment. Don't hang on. Trust that there is another beautiful inhale coming to you.

E As the belly contracts, exhale any old emotion that might be present.

S Stay open while the exhale completes the previous moment of your life. The exhales invite us to let go and release. Stay open while the energy is leaving you, and resist the need to hang on to your story for now.

Today's Practice Notes

_____

_____

_____

_____

Day 4

*"Mental balance is the perfected space between
mental strength and mental flexibility."*

— ED HARROLD

THE WAY WE START AND END our day—our twenty-four-hour cycle—is critical to our connection to something out there that's greater than ourselves. Mother Nature's inherent power directs the rise and fall of the tides, the dance of the sun and moon, the turning of the seasons and the length of our days and nights. When we tune our awareness in to this force, we become deeply aware, perceiving the bigger picture of our short time on Earth.

Breathe slowly. This slows down your perception of man-made time and brings you into Mother Nature's time. Creating more space in time in the morning sets you up for a day with less stress.

What you're thinking and feeling early in the day sets your nervous system's tempo for the rest of the day. Let go of yesterday and allow a day of new potential to arise deep inside your heart. No need to replay yesterday—today is the day your dreams can come true.

Allow yourself to wake and begin to engage the day before the sunrise. Start slowly, not rushing thoughts, emotions, or actions. Choosing to merge with energies greater than yourself through a daily ritual of self-care and mindfulness establishes a strong, heart-centered foundation on which to build the rest of your day. As life throws curveballs and presents challenges, you can remain in a state of peace and equanimity, making informed choices from your center, navigating with a sense of ease, possessing a confidence and knowing that *all* will be okay.

When you're startled awake by an alarm, hit the snooze button three times and then fly out of bed and scramble to make it out the door in time, you end up forsaking self-care for "it'll have to do." You begin the day on a crumbling foundation. This is how we set ourselves up for knee-jerk reactivity, irritability, and a daylong game of catch-up. But as we begin to discipline our mind in healthy ways, these harried days become fewer and farther between and we begin to understand and integrate the amazing benefits of beginning the day in a loving ritual of self-care. It's one of the greatest gifts we can give to ourselves and to others. The more we care for ourselves, the more able we are to care for others.

Close the day with a ritual of gratitude for what you've experienced, taking time to hold yourself with the utmost love, respect, and appreciation for having the courage to show up. Take the time to bring any heightened emotions down and into balance before falling asleep. Review the choices you made today with heartfelt awareness, not ego-based judgment.

Life is tough. You're tougher. Relax your body and your mind. Instead of worrying about tomorrow, be grateful that the sun brings the opportunity of a new day.

☀ *Today's Practice*

Diaphragmatic Breathing Step 1:

In today's practice, you'll be expanding your abdomen *before* your rib cage. When you inhale, imagine you're filling a beautiful vase from the bottom up. As you inhale through the nose, let your belly swell away from your spine. Rest your hands on your belly as you practice—this will help your brain adapt to mastering this technique. You might like doing this seated or while lying on your back. Skillful engagement of the diaphragm is paramount to moving blocked energy and stalling the aging process at the cellular level.

Now that you've practiced expanding your belly as you breathe, you'll allow the breath to expand your rib cage and fill it up to your collarbone. Gently place your hands on your ribs; inhale, filling the belly first; and allow the lower ribs to drop down and the middle and upper ribs to expand like gills. Practice this several times, and then several times more without your hands on your ribs. Now you have it. The complete inhale: belly first, lower ribs second, middle to upper ribs last. Notice the effects this has on your body and mind as you practice throughout the day.

You can practice this on your back, in a chair, on a meditation cushion, or in a light cardio routine. The idea here is to get the brain to remember this form of breathing as quickly as possible without straining.

P Set new breathing patterns in motion with compassion. Practice each time you become aware of your breath.

I Stay in beginner's mind, always learning something new.

E As your diaphragm muscle becomes more effective, imagine you're washing old emotions from the upper gut on a washboard.

S Consciously allow the mind's eye and ear to get information from the heart. First, feel with your heart. Second, think with your brain. Relax your face. Eyes can be closed or open. As you inhale, the energy and awareness move down your spine, and as you exhale, energy moves up.

Today's Practice Notes

_____

_____

_____

_____

Day 5

"Who looks outside, dreams; who looks inside, awakes."

— CARL JUNG

A PERSONAL SELF-CARE RITUAL at the beginning and end of each day is paramount to the evolving human being. Through self-care, we learn techniques that allow the body and mind to work at higher and higher levels of awareness without creating unhealthy stress. It's our time every day to connect with ourselves on every level and acknowledge that our body is a conduit for our entire experience in our lifetime. It all begins and ends with a breath.

Your self-care ritual can be as simple as practicing conscious, controlled respiration, along with an Ayurvedic self-massage called abhyanga, which oxygenates and stimulates the body through the skin. Abhyanga increases circulation, detoxifies the tissues, and boosts immune function, all while soothing the mind, which, in turn, brings that conscious, nutrient-rich breath deeper into the body. It's simple and powerful!

The skin is the largest organ in the body. Keeping the skin moist and humid allows us to move more energy in the body and raise the alkaline levels. When it's warm and humid, conditions often associated with spring and summer, it's easy to move the body and thoughts are bountiful. When it's cold and dry, conditions associated with autumn and winter, it becomes difficult to move the body, and the mind has a harder time coming up with new ideas and making informed choices. When you massage your body with warm oils, either before or after bathing, your skin remains moist and the inside of the body begins to "think" that it's the warm and humid seasons of spring and summer and responds accordingly. We want to give our bodies the balance they need through the change of seasons while coming into the teachings of the seasons themselves. Spring is a time of birth, regeneration, the return of the light. Summer is a time of action and activity. Autumn is the time of the harvest and a time of preparing the body and mind for winter, which is the time of introspection, quiet, slow movement, and integration of the experiences throughout the year.

☀ Today's Practice

Ocean-Sound Breath Technique:

While breathing through your nostrils, slightly constrict your throat, making your breath sound like the ocean. The shrinking of the airway passage allows your abdominal diaphragm to work harder than normal, and this resistance strengthens the muscle. The diaphragm plays a major role in removing wastes and raising energy in the body without raising heart rate or putting a major strain on autonomic function. Contracting your larynx creates warm heat in the throat, which removes excess mucus, phlegm, and fat from your windpipe area. Your mind also benefits from ocean-sound breath. As it investigates the sound and its "tone," your mind shifts from being reactive to being receptive. This allows you to put witnessing before judging, compassion before competition, and observing before labeling based on a memory of a past event.

Bring your palm to mouth, close your eyes, exhale through your mouth, and pretend your palm is a mirror that you're trying to fog. Use your mind to identify exactly where the sound is coming from in the throat. Do this for several mouth exhales. Then close your mouth, open your eyes if you wish and practice making the sound only while exhaling through your nose. Do this throughout the day. Don't worry if you don't get it right away. Sometimes it takes a few days. Keep practicing!

P Become aware of the muscles around your throat, and make subtle, gentle, and moderate contractions around your windpipe. Repeat, repeat, repeat.

I Notice your level of mental presence. What is your level of connection to a deeper thinking of past, present, and future?

E When you make the ocean sound, your brain will allow the wisdom of the heart to merge with all the previous choices of the mind. Turn inward with the ocean sound.

S Using ocean-sound breath allows spirit into the "choosing process" of who you really are (as opposed to who you thought you were).

Today's Practice Notes

Day 6

*"Whoever is careless with the truth in small matters
cannot be trusted with important matters."*

— ALBERT EINSTEIN

YOUR BODY IS A SACRED GIFT from the universe. What you choose to do with this gift is your responsibility. As with tending to our garden or keeping our homes clean, treating your body like a gift sometimes requires strong maintenance habits. We create and re-create ourselves every second of our life; every moment counts. Nothing escapes the Universe's eye; it sees and hears everything.

Human awareness is physical, mental, emotional, and spiritual. Every thought is a wave of vibration and frequency that travels through you and out into space. We have no lasting secrets. Everything rises to the surface eventually. The universe maintains a balance but, as individuals, we often make choices through low awareness that upset our equilibrium. As you regain your balance, try to remember that you're safe and trust in the process. Even if you're in pain, that's only one small part of you. Most parts of you are pain-free, complete, and lovable. But pain can make us forget the better aspects of ourselves.

As your breath assists you in bringing yourself back into balance, you'll feel a deep release of the old pattern and it will be replaced with a higher awareness or healthier choice. Since there are no eternal secrets, have the courage to tell the truth and fill your mind with your heart's guidance even if it temporarily hurts. Healing and transformation come from interacting with our heart's wisdom and holding ourselves accountable for that knowing by making conscious, heart-centered choices.

❋ *Today's Practice*

Apply counting to your breathing practice today. Not only does this allow you to track and improve breathing patterns, but it also keeps the mind present in the experience. So we're training the body *and* the mind.

Count the number of seconds it takes you to fill your lungs. Strive to make your exhale take twice as long as your inhale. If you're inhaling for a count of three, try exhaling for a count of six. We want to improve the exhale because the exhale is the parasympathetic response. And we want to improve a relaxed inhale to lessen the charge around the sympathetic response.

Remember the ocean-sound breath from Day 5. Today we'll use the ocean sound and combine it with the diaphragmatic breath through the nostrils. Two techniques now become one. This should be practiced as much as you can until it occurs without your trying to make it happen. We want the blending of the techniques to eventually happen without our thinking about it.

P	Taking physical control of the exhale process and breaking it down is a major step in bringing your energy centers back into balance.
I	The mind loves the exhales if you trust that it's okay to relax, to feel, to be you. When we relax and slow down, we can see our lives clearly. Fears hide strengths and pain hides pleasure.
E	As your story is transformed and old emotions are dissolved, trust that your new story is an improvement and that your best days are just in front of you.

S The process of "remembering" requires that we remove our childhood imprints. I remember many times when I said "yes" to something when I was young but didn't have the personal awareness that "no" was the right choice at the time. There were also many times when I thought "no" but said "yes." As you practice life with breath, the old "no" will turn into a new "yes," and the old "yes" will now be a firm "no."

Today's Practice Notes

Day 7

*"Unexpressed emotions will never die. They are buried
alive and will come forth later in uglier ways."*

— SIGMUND FREUD

LOVE YOUR BELLY. Emotions live in the belly. It's your connection to the feminine principle. Feminine is creative; it's not afraid to shake things up today for a better tomorrow. There's so much more to the intelligence of the belly than "what it looks like." In the quest for six-pack abs, we've cut ourselves off from one of our greatest sources of information. It doesn't really matter what your belly looks like—what really matters is what your belly *feels* like. The belly is the master feeler, and feelings don't lie. They're a raw, natural form of emotional intelligence. Believe it or not, we're all really good at emotional intelligence—we just have to pause and remember that feelings are messages that must be witnessed, not judged.

When our belly is tight, our thoughts are restricted. Relaxing the belly relaxes the mind. When the mind is untethered, we can become creative again. It's so hard to create anything new in our mind when the belly is too tight to think, stressing out the heart. This weakens our immune system over time, and restricted thoughts and feelings begin to accumulate. When we can access those thoughts and feelings from the gut, we find a new source of information available to us. This creates high self-esteem, confidence, and peace.

Nasal breathing allows the diaphragm muscle to press downward on the inhale. Strengthening the diaphragm keeps energy moving in the belly. The abdomen receives a huge massage or wave of energy. This strengthens the digestive process and allows us to quickly eliminate the past, letting go of the old and making way for the new.

Don't judge your belly for what it looks like, but be aware of what it feels like at any moment. It reads the external environment and lets you know if you're safe and if the people around you are sincere. Feelings don't lie; thoughts do. Your belly always tells the truth and never wastes energy on mindless fantasies. Spend more time listening to your belly—it can be a great friend.

❊ Today's Practice

While walking today, apply yesterday's technique of counting the breath and making your exhale twice as long as your inhale. There are two ways to administer the counting: If you're a left-brain person or your profession is very left-brain-dominant, I suggest you count your strides so that you're connecting mind with body; if you're a right-brain person or in a creative profession, you might want to count with the rhythm your feet make while touching the earth to create the experience from the ground up through the body. I like to count from the body, not the head. I'm a kinesthetic learner, so it's perfect for me. This practice will become a walking meditation.

> **P** With each step, mindfully connect the breath with the movement. Feel your feet grounding you with each step. Heel to ball joint. While the foot is going down to the ground, try to draw the arch up under the bones of your foot. Practice this while you walk; it's a great technique for activating the skeletal muscles of your lower body. This creates optimal balance, power, and circulation.

I When you inhale, mentally *send* your intention to the creative force of the universe. What do you want to occur in this moment? What are you creating? Is it love or fear?

E To think safer thoughts, we must first *feel* safe. Feel your exhale creating safety, relaxing you, removing stress.

S We are limitless beings with self-imposed limits. Be abundant as you expand beyond your past limits.

Today's Practice Notes

Day 8

"If I have ever made any valuable discoveries, it has been owing more to patient attention, than to any other talent."

— WILLIAM SHAKESPEARE

L EARNING THE SKILL OF ATTENTION is one of the gifts of a daily breathing practice. Refining mental states of attention is key to balancing energy and awareness. Where are you placing your attention on a daily basis? Where we can have trust, there will be truth, and where there's truth, there's peace. When my clients talk about what's missing in their lives and relationships, they often say there isn't any peace or there isn't enough peace. That perception can be traced back to not trusting themselves or their choices. If you trace it back even further, you'll find that, in general, there's an absence of truth in their lives.

Our perception of having power or being powerless plays a huge role in our trust level and in how much or little we trust our states of awareness. But, with practice, we can learn to trust the wisdom of our belly. By listening to the solar plexus, right below the heart, we can get more information and make more informed choices. Trusting the divine wisdom of the belly requires you to refine how you see yourself and how you allow the world to view you. Trusting that you're okay and will remain safe is the key to this step, along with slow, conscious breathing.

There is your truth and then there's the Universe's truth. If there's separation between them, returning to wholeness will require healing. But facing this can be difficult because we fear it will hurt and we've been conditioned to believe we should avoid pain at all costs. People often equate pain with suffering, but this isn't so. Pain is a message, a teacher. Suffering is a choice.

When you're in a conflict, observe your thoughts and invite yourself to explore the space between being so right that you couldn't possibly be wrong and being completely wrong. This will broaden your perspective. Also, question and explore your need to be right. When our heart is aligned with universal truth, our need to be right dissolves along with our attachments and fears. This allows our desire to act for the higher good to emerge and blossom.

When we're peaceful, we're at our full power. Releasing our small truths and attachments and embracing the massive universal truths of love, compassion, and right relationships is an amazing feeling. This is a real lifting of the monkey off our back, and we become lighter on all levels, walk a little taller, and stop taking ourselves so seriously. There's liberation in letting go of the need to be right about everything all the time.

☀ Today's Practice

Four-Part Breath with Ocean Sound:

Today, we'll combine everything you learned during the first week into a flowing exercise. Breathe through your nose with a soft ocean sound in the throat. Keep your facial muscles as relaxed as you can. Release and relax your eyes, and release and relax your lower jaw. Inhale slowly, and then pause for a moment and notice the quality of your mind. Exhale through your nose with an ocean sound, and then pause and notice the quality of your mind.

When you're ready for a compassionate challenge, allow your exhale to be longer than the inhale. But please don't rush the inhale. If you feel short of breath, don't exhale quite as long or don't pause after the exhale. Once your cardiovascular system catches up with your nervous system, resume the four-part breathing practice.

FOUR-PART BREATH TECHNIQUE

Step 1 Count your inhale.

   Tip: Continue inhaling until there's a gentle lift of the upper ribs toward your lower jaw.

Step 2 Hold your inhale in for one count.

   Tip: Relax and let a gentle pressure build from the inside out.

Step 3 Exhale for the same length of time as your inhale.

   Tip: "Bleed" the air out of the lungs using the ocean sound while controlling the length, depth, and pace.

Step 4 Hold your out breath for one count. This is the most challenging part.

   Tip: Stay calm and relaxed. Don't panic. There is stale air in the alveolar sacs in your lungs that gets used when you hold your breath out. Don't strain.

Also, make a mental note not to rush the pace of your next inhale. If you find that you're rushing the inhale, skip the hold-out round of your sequence for a round or two and then gently try to introduce the holding-out period again. Remember, patience and practice without being competitive are key to growth.

P   Feel a relaxed, calm rush of energy rise during the internal breath retentions.

I   When breath is held in, watch the brain, heart, and mind merge into one pointed awareness or direction.

E   When your breath is held out, toxic emotional debris will be removed from the nervous system.

S   We create space in the mind during internal retentions. We begin to see that we are choosing how much or how little we allow into our life.

Today's Practice Notes

Day 9

*"Be a lifelong learner. Learn one new thing
a day, 365 new things a year. This learning
keeps us expanding, happy and light."*

— ED HARROLD

B OTTOM-UP LEARNING IS AN awareness-based model. Learning from the feet up to the belly, heart, and head, we embody the learning. It's awareness-based because it's been experienced in the body, not just in the mind. We're constantly learning and evolving. Learning is the foundation of our vitality and vibrancy.

I love learning and becoming more aware of the big picture of my life. But there's an old part of me that likes to view life and my choices through the narrowest of lenses and resists personal growth and change. I've learned that to see the bigger picture, we have to feel physically safe. When we feel safe in body, the brain will allow expansion in the mind, creating new awareness.

Consider what most of us experienced in school. We sat at a desk and the teacher relayed information by talking and using visual aids. We were expected to learn by using only our auditory and visual channels. We had very little opportunity to learn kinesthetically—with our body, through movement, touch, and direct experience. Those of us who were primarily kinesthetic learners were often shamed and treated as if we were stupid or lazy. What story did we learn to tell about those experiences? How many of us grew up thinking we were unintelligent or incapable, square pegs being shoved into round holes?

Regardless of our past experience, we can expand our awareness and extract information from consciousness with increasing skill through kinesthetic experience and learning directly through the body (feeling/knowing) as well as with our eyes and ears. As we develop these skills, we receive more information about our environment, first rooting and grounding the body through the nervous system and then opening to the full range of our sensory perception and beyond. We make more informed choices in life when we feel balanced between our emotions and our intellect.

✳ Today's Practice

Breathe in slowly through your nose, and at the top of the inhale pause for two seconds while holding your breath in. Exhale slowly through your nose and pause for two seconds at the end of the exhale while holding your breath out. This is the basic four-part breath. If you rush the process of exhale or inhale, you agitate the nervous or cardiovascular systems. You may feel a little heat when you practice this technique.

1. Slowly inhale

2. Pause, holding breath in for two seconds

3. Slowly exhale

4. Pause, holding breath out for two seconds

5. Repeat

While practicing the four-part breath, contract your abdominal muscles when pausing. In yoga, this is the second bandha, or lock. Yogis know of a deep well of bottomless energy stored in the belly that the mental ego controls. When we use energy stored in the belly, the body releases life-force energy that can evolve the ego beyond our current perceptions.

Creating a contraction in the abdominal muscles allows the body's fire to rise and create heat in the digestive organs.

These organs are sensitive, emotional areas where we hold old patterns and behaviors. Burning a stronger flame in the lower abdomen clears the way for moving forward in life.

NOTE: You will notice that your heart rate goes a little higher when you contract the abdominal muscles than when you don't. If the pace of your heart rate scares you, do the squeezing technique every other breath until you're ready to do it with each breath.

P When you pause the breathing, gently engage the muscles from your pelvic floor to your solar plexus.

I If you see an opportunity to go deeper into your mind, do this. Don't be afraid, and don't bring your ego.

E Emotions control thoughts. The breathing and retention clear out all the old "stuff." It's an emotional cleanse.

S Stay present today. Don't spiritualize your ego. Enjoy the heightened awareness without attachment. It's like looking at something beautiful without having to own it.

Today's Practice Notes

Day 10

"During the time of stress, the "fight-or-flight"
response is on and the self-repair mechanism is disabled.
It is then when we say that the immunity of the
body goes down and the body is exposed to the risk
for disease. Meditation activates relaxation,
when the sympathetic nervous system is turned
off and the parasympathetic nervous system is
turned on, and natural healing starts."

— ANNIE WILSON, EFFECT OF MEDITATION ON
CARDIOVASCULAR HEALTH, IMMUNITY & BRAIN FITNESS

TODAY'S PRACTICE, CALLED ALTERNATE nostril breathing, allows us to drop into a meditative state very quickly. Conscious breathing prepares the nervous system for the many beneficial effects of a meditation practice. Many people are disappointed if they don't receive the gifts of meditation right away. Sitting daily and engaging in a pranayama practice before meditation allows a softening to take place by giving the mind something to watch. That helps us to sit quietly and begin the process of silencing the voices in our head.

Inhaling through the right nasal channel feeds the left, masculine, solar, directive side of the brain. Inhaling through the left nasal channel feeds the right, feminine, lunar, receptive side of the brain. The left brain is home to our perception of time. The right brain is home to our perception of space. Transcending our perception that we're bound and limited by time will lower our stress level and open our minds to new creative thoughts and solutions. Time is always on our side and time is all we have. Slowing our perception of time begins with alternate nostril breathing. The calming release of serotonin balances the fast-paced rhythm of adrenaline.

Scientific research indicates that when we're in a meditative state, the left brain is enveloped by the right as awareness enters our mind's eye. The normal pulls of the left prefrontal cortex into fear or insecurity states dissolve into the activity of the right brain. We think less. The stories around our stress-filled life in the left brain dissolve like a mirage in the desert. When we create more space in our mind and bring our brain and heart into a synchronicity known as physiological coherence, we become fully aware of being calm and fearless as our natural state. When entering the space for the first time, allow a sense of wonder and just witness what happens without emotional attachment or analysis. Where attachment and the thinking mind are present, there is no meditation. Surrender your will in that space. You're in God's hands now.

✴ Today's Practice

Alternate Nostril Breathing:

First, completely relax everything from the inside out for five long, slow, deep breaths and get yourself fully present, in the moment and awake.

You can practice alternate nostril breathing while sitting, standing, or walking. Curl in the first two fingers of your right hand. Place your thumb outside your right nostril and your ring finger outside your left nostril. Let your pinky extend so that it's not in the way. Use your thumb to close off your right nostril channel, inhale up the left nostril channel, close the left nostril with your ring finger, release your thumb, and exhale out your right nasal channel. Inhale up your right nasal channel, close the right nasal channel with your thumb, release your ring finger, and exhale out your left nasal channel. Repeat. Use ocean-sound breath to slow your breathing rate until you master this.

NOTE: As you practice, consciously relax your eyes, mouth, lips, and jaw.

P   Trace the path of the inhales and exhales to the opposite side of the prefrontal cortex. (i.e., left nostril inhale to right side of prefrontal cortex. Right nostril inhale to left prefrontal cortex.)

I   Visualize a crossing of the breath at the bridge of your nose and brow. This crossing of the breath, which would look like an X or a crossroads if you could see it, helps synchronize the two sides of your prefrontal cortex so they work as one.

E   During this exercise, negative emotions will not have the same pull on your awareness.

S   This *crossroads* is the first bridge to using the whole brain. This whole-brain thinking and awareness are critical for seeing beyond where we've been and seeing where we're going.

Today's Practice Notes

_____

_____

_____

_____

Day 11

*"Cooking is great, but the meal that has been
prepared for you with love is the best."*

— STEPHEN RICHARDS

AFTER CONSCIOUS BREATHING or pranayama, one of the most important tools in energizing and balancing your life is conscious eating. Pray before each meal, taking a moment to honor the meal itself and how it got from Mother Earth to your table. Instead of unconsciously racing through your meals, eat slowly, putting down the knife and fork to chew consciously, truly tasting your food and mindfully taking it into your body. Food is potential energy, fuel—that's it. It's designed to keep you alive, not to repress difficult emotions or celebrate pleasure.

Mealtime is a sacred time. It's when we slow down, relax, and reflect on greater things. We rest our minds for a moment and take a breath or two, giving thanks for the meal and all the work it took to bring it to our plates. The sunlight, soil, and rain, the farmer, the trucker who brought the food to market and everyone in between. So much energy and effort is expended in preparing food for us, from the earth to the table, that it seems that we would have more awareness and gratitude for the whole process. Instead of complaining about grocery shopping, we have the opportunity to consider how hard complete strangers worked to bring that food to market for us. There's an opportunity for gratitude in everything we experience.

So, beginning today, give mealtime the focus it deserves. Make eating a wholly conscious act, sitting with good posture, feet on ground, spine erect, face and eyes relaxed. No distractions, silence or soft conversation, no loud voices or excess emotion. Proper digestion begins in the mouth with lots of chewing, breaking down energy for the stomach, and with the proper gratitude. Smile when you're eating. Enjoy the gift.

Cultivate a proper mental attitude of gratitude for the food and the energy of the earth. It takes a long time for Mother Nature to create food for us. When eating, enjoy the bounty of the earth and give thanks to nature and any animals that have given their life for you to live another day. Pray and lovingly energize the molecules that make up the meal. Bring the full power of the Universe to your plate. Notice the portion size and be aware that your stomach is only the size of your fist. Ask yourself, "Is taking in this food affirming something my body needs, or is it my ego trying to weaken my body?" Think about why you chose the food that's on your plate. Are you eating from emotion or an inner knowing of what fuel your body requires in the present moment to get you to the next moment?

☀ Today's Practice

While you're eating, inhale and exhale through your nose as slowly as you can. Be mindful of chewing, the taste of the food, and the texture. Chew your food thoroughly. This will aid in the digestion, elimination, and assimilation of your food.

P   Slow the pace of your breathing to fully taste the flavors of your food. Slow breathing also helps with breaking down the food to be recooked in the stomach.

I   Relax the mind, release old thoughts and be grateful for this meal, this bite, this energy that Mother Earth has worked so hard to bring to your body.

E Food is like sex. There are many thousands of nerve endings in and around the mouth. Give yourself this simple pleasure.

S Imagine the journey your food has taken to reach your mouth. From the planting of the seed, through its growth and harvest and on to the grocer for your home and table. Consider the many hands and forces that helped to make this happen; the farmer, the earth, sun, wind and rain; the truck drivers or train engineers; the people who receive the food shipment at the grocery store; and the people who put in on the shelves. I love doing this simple visualization. It produces so much gratitude for people I've never even met who are in service to my life.

Today's Practice Notes

Day 12

*"Feelings come and go like clouds in a windy
sky. Conscious breathing is my anchor."*

— THICH NHAT HANH

LEARNING THE PROPER WAY TO EXHALE is a key to personal growth because of the relaxation qualities of the parasympathetic nervous system. The exhale is the signal for parasympathetic activity. The brain won't shift into transformational states if it's not calm.

In conscious breathing, we always breathe through the nose when we inhale and when we exhale. If we're feeling stressed, our sympathetic nervous system will prompt us to gasp for air or initialize a mouth breath to deliver air to the lungs more quickly. When that happens, we experience stress physiology, and our options are reduced to fight, flight, or freeze. To override this response, when you're feeling stressed, consciously hold the breath out at the end of your nasal exhale, pausing for a moment before the next inhale. Follow the pause with a slow, controlled inhale for maximum absorption of nutrient-rich air. This will give your brain what it needs to focus, make informed choices, and take the proper action. Sometimes the right action is to mindfully remove yourself from a difficult or dangerous situation, and other times the proper action is to do nothing but make space for discomfort and trust that you're truly okay. As your pranayama practice evolves, you'll be able to skillfully utilize breath holds for moments of deeper transformation throughout your life, shifting from a place of knee-jerk reaction to conscious, mindful responsiveness.

To use pranayama to control your nervous-system physiology and remain calm in less than desirable moments, start with a long, slow, deep breath and make your exhale longer than your inhale. The exhale has a cooling effect. It's a point of release, a letting go of the past moment. It's also a great indicator of how safe or unsafe we think we are. The inhale is the sympathetic aspect of our breathing pattern. When we shorten our exhale and rush our inhale, we take more breaths per minute activating a sympathetic response spiking blood pressure and heart rate. Exhaling through the nose is a major detox for all the body's systems. It allows brainwave activity to slightly slow down. It rebalances heart rates and blood pressure. It's a gateway into the back of the brain and downward-flowing energy into the pelvic bowl. And it stimulates digestion and elimination for maximum assimilation.

The exhale also prepares the body for the next inhale. When our exhale is shallow, there's stale air residue in the cells that impedes the introduction of a rich level of oxygen into the bloodstream on the next inhale. That residue robs us of the energizing arousal that oxygen-rich air provides. When the exhale is long and complete, the ability of the next inhale is amplified and magnified in the sinuses and the alveoli (air sacs in the lungs where the exchange of oxygen occurs). Saturating the blood with oxygen through conscious respiration clears the mind and takes unhealthy pressure off the heart. It also rapidly removes high levels of carbon dioxide from the bloodstream.

Holding the breath out is a tool for the mind and the body. Hold the breath out for as long as it feels comfortable without rushing the next inhale. The mind begins to engage the present moment's choices as we hold the breath out and become aware of the silence. As the next inhale stimulates the limbic system in the brain, we're presented with the opportunity to transcend fears and reclaim the time and energy they steal from us.

⚒ *Today's Practice*

Using the ocean-sound breath, completely fill your lungs and then pause. Now release 50 percent of the exhale and pause again. Then release the remaining 50 percent and pause. Do several rounds. After mastering this exhale, practice dividing the exhale into three parts instead of two. Fill your lungs to full capacity and pause. Release a third of the air from your lungs and pause. Release another third of the air and pause. Release the remaining third and pause. Practice this until it starts to feel comfortable and revisit this practice throughout the day.

Notice your personal awareness when you turn the exhale muscles on and off. Notice the meditative mind that's available to you. Practice this technique when you feel yourself starting to become anxious or stressed. You now have the tools to move yourself from a state of overwhelm to a calm, centered, meditative state.

P   Slow the inhale and enjoy releasing the exhales in smaller, bite-size pieces. It's great to practice this breathing pattern in the morning so we don't energetically burn out in the afternoon.

I   This technique quickly changes our perception of time for the better. Most folks can't keep up with time and they fall behind into stress. Stress just means you care deeply about your chance on Earth and want to do your best. As time slows down, we have greater control of the mind.

E   On the exhales, we feel. On the inhales, we think. So this technique is about feeling more than you normally allow yourself to feel.

S   When we stop censoring our heavy feelings about ourselves and life, we remember we are light, and light is limitless in its abilities.

Today's Practice Notes

_____

_____

_____

_____

Day 13

*"At first, dreams seem impossible, then
improbable, and eventually inevitable."*

— CHRISTOPHER REEVE

G OOD HEALTH STEMS FROM HARNESSING potential energy
to make better, more mindful, informed choices. All
choices serve a purpose and have value; but informed, conscious choices move us to self-growth and a deeper awareness
that we're connected to Source on every level. This occurs
consciously or unconsciously during the process of inhalation. Make it conscious so that each breath can work for your
self-development.

The inhale is vital! We must improve the process of inhalation to have the energy to change our life. It takes a ton
of energy to change course in our life. If you don't have the
energy, you'll probably quit on yourself halfway through due
to exhaustion.

How many seconds does it take to fill your lungs? Notice
that your lungs fill quickly when you inhale through your
mouth and that they fill slowly when you inhale through your
nose. Slower is better unless your life is in mortal danger. To
reach the maximum depth of breath, you want to expand and
completely fill your lungs. You can breathe more slowly and
deeply by building a strong and dynamic diaphragm muscle.
The deeper the inhale carries the oxygen into your tissues, the
healthier your blood will be, and the healthier your blood is,
the healthier you are!

The pace of the breath tells your nervous system how calm
or stressed you are. When the pace is steady and smooth, there's

an absence of stress physiology in the body, even if we're experiencing an uncomfortable moment. Smooth, steady breathing helps the heart rate to stabilize and blood pressure to normalize. Brain wave activity moves from stressful high beta waves into low beta or high alpha waves. With your breath, you can create peace in your mind, peace in your body; and peace in your world.

✵ Today's Practice

Start with ocean-sound breath and exhale longer than you inhale. Do several warm-up rounds. Now exhale and practice holding your breath out. Do several rounds of this. As you practice, the key is to not hold your breath out for so long that it impairs the length, depth, and pace of the next inhale. If that occurs, don't exhale as long or hold out as long. If you find your mind wandering, return it to the breath and begin counting the length of the inhale and exhale to give the mind something to do.

NOTE: Counting could be: Inhale four counts, exhale four counts, hold for four counts. If you want to hold the breath out for longer, don't exhale as long. If you want to exhale longer, don't hold the breath out so long.

P   Be mindful of relaxing the mind. Use breathing to add a little heat or fire, and then a little more.

I   Stay present for the shifts in the mind and the new perceptions of old thought forms.

E   Be aware of and focus on cooling your emotions and then heating them up. Watch how you feel afterward.

S Many people don't develop a spiritual practice until everything else has failed. That's okay. It's all part of your plan to heal your life, learn your lessons, get up on the medal podium again and stay there.

Today's Practice Notes

Day 14

*"Do not be anxious about tomorrow, for
tomorrow will be anxious for itself. Let the day's
own trouble be sufficient for the day."*

— JESUS

To CREATE WHAT YOU PERCEIVE TO BE GOOD in your life, you need to understand the bad. The bad isn't always as bad as we perceive it to be. Sometimes it looks bad simply because we're caught up in the same old stories. Fortunately, we can change the story any time we're ready. The truth is that every experience in life has value, whether we perceive it to be good or bad. We can learn something from everyone and every event and situation. Life *is* the practice.

We require discomfort in order to stimulate self-growth and navigate the natural cycle of change. If circumstances were wonderful all the time, we'd never grow, never move forward. And Mother Nature's patterns show us that we won't be down for long. It rains and then the sun comes out. The dark of night is always followed by the sunrise. Everything cycles. If we can get out of our own way, we'll dance through life with skill and grace. When we learn to dance, we pay attention to the lines of our body and the way we're moving through space. We're also aware of how much space we have on the dance floor or stage.

Creating or restructuring boundaries isn't just an important aspect of the dance. It's also a major step in our transformation. When we were young, we may have had low awareness and poor boundaries, trying to fit into various cliques and artificial friendships. We said yes when we should have said no. We said no when we should have said yes. As we mature, we all work to correct these choices and capitalize on the opportunities for growth. And as we grow, we move inward toward our heart.

And then something truly amazing happens.

As we deeply relax, our fears turn into great teachers that help us move beyond our old belief systems. And that process transforms fear into strength. The more we operate from our hearts, the more our strengths are authenticated on a deeper level than our egos. Our heart-centered strengths are powerful allies and illuminate darkness. If we discover that what we thought was a strength is actually a temporary crutch or device to bring instant gratification or comfort, we can release it to the Universe for recycling and explore our potential for cultivating strength from our character, values, and internal compass.

☀ *Today's Practice*

50/50 Breathing:

Using ocean-sound breath, inhale to 50 percent of your capacity and pause. Then inhale the remaining 50 percent and pause, holding the breath in. Exhale 50 percent of the air and pause, exhale the remaining 50 percent and pause. Repeat several rounds. After several rounds, allow the external retention to increase from a pause to a longer holding, but don't rush the next 50 percent inhale. Meditate on today's concepts after your breathing experience for as long as desired.

Practice this new technique and notice how quickly you can be in a meditative state of being. Try not to rush the inhales or the exhales. Refine your ocean-sound breathing again and again.

> **P** This breath, when practiced correctly and daily, allows a massive energetic shift in the body.

I   When we focus on the breath, everything else falls away and we naturally enter a meditative state of mind.

E   Balancing your high and low emotions happens almost overnight with this technique.

S   We are spirit first, body second. Life is tough, you're tougher. Life will never be easy, but this technique allows life to become less challenging.

Today's Practice Notes

Day 15

"We can easily forgive a child who is afraid of the dark;
the real tragedy of life is when men are afraid of the light."

— PLATO

TO MOVE FORWARD AND TRANSFORM old patterns is a conscious choice for liberation and empowerment. To obtain or cultivate something new, we must surrender or let go of the old that no longer serves us. It's a simple matter of creating space. It's impossible to hold on to old paradigms and successfully shift into new ones. Thankfully, transformation can be a natural process as we breathe ourselves awake and find that we can easily and gratefully let go of all that no longer serves our greater purpose.

Consciously evolving requires disciplining our thoughts and feelings and having faith in the work. It means honoring the journey, even the days that don't feel good. When the negative or critical self-talk begins, remain mindful and centered and tap into the unchanging still point within you. That's where you'll find truth and light. Take a breath and give yourself a moment to witness the thoughts and self-defeating chatter. Then choose a healthy action that's based in self-love, forgiveness, and deep, honest inquiry.

People who understand the deeper workings of manifestation know that thoughts form intention and that intention is more powerful and magnetic than any individual thought. We can form intentions that support us in pursuing our life's purpose, and we can also form intentions that hinder our growth and progress. When we form intentions that are meant to support our purpose, we manifest what will benefit us most. The key is creating context for what you truly desire and deciding how much energy and time you can invest in creating or attracting it. Everyone wants life to improve, but nobody wants to change. We need to find value in all the resources we have now, instead of focusing on what we don't have, shutting down and tuning out.

How Change Happens for Adults:

1. Notice the opportunity to have a different perception of an old thought form, mood, or behavior.

2. Decide how much you want this new awareness to integrate a change or perception in your subconscious mind.

3. Decide what you're willing to surrender to the Universe that which no longer serves you.

4. Change takes place.

5. Repeat.

6. Smile, if applicable. ☺

Consider how you can achieve what you desire with the least amount of force. You don't want to create a ton of stress and pain for yourself, coworkers, and family members. It takes time to transform an intention into a physical manifestation, so keep your faith and your intention strong. A weak intention is nothing but a wish; but strong, focused intention enables you to consciously cocreate your life. Set your intention, hold your head high with your new awareness, and trust that the Universe heard your prayer. Now put one foot in front of the other. Remember the old saying, "God helps those who help themselves"?

Don't judge whether the Universe is cocreating with you based on your human perception of time. The Universe isn't based in our time-space continuum. The Universe is based in energy and collective consciousness. The larger, more extensive, or detailed the desired manifestation is, the more time and energy it will require. Set yourself up for success by maintaining your pranayama practice, keeping your mind clear and your body healthy. Just like any other skill, learning to manifest takes time and practice, and it can also take time to fully trust the process. When your faith wavers or you have doubts, align your awareness with the universal consciousness and remember that you're protected, supported, and loved.

☀ *Today's Practice*

Four-Part Breath Variation:

Using ocean-sound breath, inhale and count how long it takes you to fill your lungs without strain. Hold for twice as long as it took you to inhale. Exhale for the same count as the inhale and pause. Do several rounds, gradually increasing the count of the exhale and the count of holding the exhale out, until they match the count of the inhale.

No matter what your count is, the ratio for four-part breathing is:

Inhale for five counts. Slow-motion inhale.

Hold for ten counts. Relax and feel yourself expanding on every level.

Exhale for five counts. Exhale a little faster than you normally would.

Hold for five counts. This will be the hardest part.

The formula could change, but it's all based on the length of the inhale.

For example:

8/16/8/8

7/14/7//7

4/8/4/4

3/6/3/3

After practicing four-part breathing, meditate on your experience for as long as possible, seated or walking.

P   Strengthening our respiratory muscles takes unhealthy pressure off our cardiovascular organs, giving us a huge advantage.

I   The more oxygen the brain senses (which is a sign of a healthy cardiovascular system), the more dopamine and serotonin it releases and the more happy thoughts we have.

E   This exercise churns and purifies old, unhealthy emotional behaviors.

S   You come from light. You are light now. You will return to this light. Be light today.

Today's Practice Notes

Day 16

*"The goal of spiritual practice is full recovery,
and the only thing you need to recover
from is a fractured sense of self."*

— MARIANNE WILLIAMSON

A S WE BEGIN TO SEE THAT WE'RE powerful beyond our wildest dreams, it can get a little scary. Take a moment to appreciate the innate power and wisdom we were all born with. Life isn't meant to be a constant struggle. It's our birthright to be happy, safe, and fully loved.

Most of us strongly connect with our fears and experience a lot of uncertainty. It's almost as if we have to figure out what we don't want in order to identify what we do want. It's learning through the process of elimination. This is pretty counterintuitive, isn't it? No other animal on the planet uses the process of elimination to figure out what it wants. Because we're at the top of the food chain, our process of self-discovery is forgiving and gives us many chances to grow and transform. Each new day brings another opportunity to heal, change, and create the exact life we want. Embracing the opportunity is as easy as waking up and setting an intention to be more compassionate *today* to yourself and others. Whatever you require or desire, you can create if you're willing to give it the time and energy.

When you work with the energetic, emotional heart, you become confident in your skills, balance your emotions, become less reactive and more confident in your choices, and develop higher self-esteem. Take things one breath at a time, one awareness at a time, one choice at a time. What's the rush? Life will be over soon enough. You are liberated. You are God/consciousness in a body. You are not your personality—you're a soul having a physical experience.

⁑ *Today's Practice*

Start by reviewing the alternate nostril breathing from Day 10. Do several rounds. After getting steady and quiet, start to add a pause after each inhale before you switch to the other nasal channel. Continue with several rounds. When you pause, gaze deeply into your inner world. Tap into that blank space during the pausing period. This is one of my favorites. Try to create what appears to be blank space in your mind's eye or ear. Go toward the blank space without straining. Or let the blank space organically come toward you like a magnet. Be still and let your awareness become "nondoing," just being.

NOTE: Don't rush your breathing with adding the pause after the inhale. Exhale slowly, controlling the length and pace of exhale with ocean-sound breath.

> **P** You are repattering how the energy of the breath enters the prefrontal cortex. When both nostrils are open and breathing equally, everything is in a state of "flow" (or "in the zone").

> **I** Blend feeling and thought as one awareness.

> **E** During this exercise, emotional intelligence is cleared and amplified. There isn't pain or pleasure. Everything is energy and awareness *without* the peaks and valleys of previous success or failure.

S This is the beginning of the end of the old you. It's also the beginning of reclaiming peace, compassion, kindness, and everything else that love is made of.

Today's Practice Notes

_____

_____

_____

_____

Day 17

"Our past is a plus, not a minus. If you can't
see or feel the past in a positive light, don't go there
mentally today. Just because you don't have
the answer you prefer today, doesn't mean you
won't have it tomorrow if you don't shut down
the process and surf the waves of your life."

— ED HARROLD

WHEN WE'RE YOUNG WE HAVE so much energy, but we don't have the awareness. As we move through the experiences of life, our energy levels drop but our awareness levels should expand. To begin a bright, light future, we need to become accountable for everything we do, say, and think. The future begins today. We can't change the past, but we can change our emotions into new understanding, and we can heal the wounds we've covered up and tried to ignore.

If you're willing to identify only with the good parts of your past, you're missing out on half your life. All of us make mistakes. Everyone's done something they're not proud of, but when we harbor shame, we give it the power to limit how we think, what we believe, and how we live. Shame is an energy thief, but you can thwart its efforts by shining a light on the roots of your shame and objectively examining them. As long as the roots remain buried, you feed them with the deep belief that you deserve to feel ashamed and aren't worthy of love exactly as you are. Shame makes you feel heavy and dense, whereas love, forgiveness, and gratitude lift you up and make you feel light and bright. The breathing practices will help you to remember that you can transcend the limiting beliefs you've acquired through direct experience or influence.

Investigate the roots of your beliefs without guilt. View your choices with the open mind of an explorer, and take responsibility for your role in how everything played out. How we perceive the past is important. Hindsight is 20/20, but we can still get caught up in blame and needing to be right. Holding ourselves accountable to something greater than our individual self expands our awareness.

We stop feeling like we're victims of life's circumstances when we see that everything is happening for our benefit, even the difficult, heartbreaking stuff. It all has value. When we choose to remain present, we don't allow strong emotional charges to steal moments and right action from us. Instead, we start to use these challenging experiences to increase our awareness, learn, and grow. The more of the big picture we can see, the greater our belief that everything was, is, and will be okay.

⚵ *Today's Practice*

Incremental Breathing:

Using the ocean-sound breath, inhale to 50 percent capacity, pause, and inhale to full capacity. Pause, and then exhale in four parts, at a rate of 25 percent each time. I like my exhale to be twice as long as my inhale, and incremental breathing allows this to happen in a powerful way. It's a simple technique: Inhale in two segments and exhale in four segments. Play with the length of the pauses.

When you practice this with great awareness, it will quickly take you deep into your heart. This is great for relaxing after work and before going to sleep.

> **P**   As the breathing becomes refined, so does everything else in the body. This refinement is crucial

to reclaiming the heart's original blueprint of your purpose.

I   Every time you practice, notice the brain fog, distraction, or confusion dissolving in your mind and in your thoughts.

E   Each emotion has a seed of intelligence. Capturing its raw intelligence is like learning a new skill. Breathing in fractions of one-quarter at a time allows us to trace information back to its source.

S   The four-part breath is about balance and the number four as a spiritual number is a calming force. This technique is setting in motion a balanced perception of a spiritual life, which is living a peaceful life despite the appearance of anything but peace everywhere you look.

Today's Practice Notes

_____

_____

_____

_____

Day 18

*"Our choices have consequences.
We can't see all the ways it can go right,
and you can't see all the ways not right.
Slow down your breath, and be
grounded in your choices."*

— WENDY HARROLD

M Y WIFE AND LIFE PARTNER has a wonderful awareness that our choices are huge. We *always* have a choice, even when it seems we have none. The more information we have, the more choices we have. And the more choices we have, the more successful we'll be with our healing and transformation. So being informed is huge, and that goes for what's going on in our environment and inside our minds and bodies.

Without choices, nothing would ever change in our lives. We'd make the same choices at age thirty that we made at age fifteen. So the choice process is very important. I work with many types of people in many platforms. At first they want everything in their life to change but don't change anything; no new thoughts, no new habits, no new behaviors, nothing new! They don't realize that choices are the key to changing old perceptions, old awareness, and old memories. Believe me, nothing will change until there are more choices or options for moving forward. Folks who don't have any choice are suffering much more than those who have choices and options for dealing with life's challenges.

To correct our illusions and see the truth, we need to be able to tell the difference between the critical, egotistical voice in our head and the heart-centered inner voice of knowing and detachment.

When we fully explore a thought, when we sit for a breath and feel the thought in our belly, something amazing happens to our perception of that thought. If there's an unhealthy aspect of the thought, our belly will let us know. The body won't lie, so we become instantly aware of being attached to a particular outcome or of honoring our higher Self. The belly lets us know whether a thought is born from fear or from love.

When we use the centering belly together with a conscious heart, our thoughts and feelings gain clarity and we develop a deeper understanding of our current level of awareness. This is an important part of healing because every organ in the body resonates with a dominant emotion. The liver resonates with anger, the lungs with grief, the stomach with stress and the kidneys with depression. The heart is true love without attachment. Living from the heart is the highest calling, and while it's almost impossible for us to do this for an extended time, it's the lightest and brightest of the human experience. It also requires a major commitment of time, energy, and resources.

When our organs relay information about our experience to our mind via the brain, we can become more deeply aware of the creative potential that a new moment can hold for us. When we become aware of the beliefs we're holding in the mind and the trauma we're holding in our cells, we can begin the process of healing and release, moving deeper into awareness of the whole and away from the illusion of separation. We never forget those healing moments of awareness. We experience them in both the body and the mind, and they leave an imprint on our heart, creating catharsis.

Emptying the organs of mucus and fats is the first step of transformation. When the internal walls of our organs are free of wastes, less energy is required for digestion. That new energy is sent to the brain, and we have more energy for neuroplasticity and new awareness of old thoughts in the mind. Slow your breath, smile, and relax. Live with your entire self, not just your head or your body. You're doing great, probably a lot better than you give yourself credit for. Don't be so hard on yourself.

✳ Today's Practice

Four-Part Breath, building muscles of exhale:

Using ocean-sound breath, count your inhale and hold your breath in for the same length of time. Double the count of your inhale, and make your exhale that long. Then pause at the end of the exhale and return to the inhale.

The counting might look like this:

Inhale for five counts. Relax and feel the fresh energy entering your inner world.

Hold for five counts. Feel the inhale's qualities going deeper inside you.

Exhale for ten counts. Try to exhale in slow motion, really bleeding the carbon dioxide out of the lungs.

Hold breath out for two counts. Stay calm, with good posture on all levels. Gradually increase the counts that you're holding the breath out until it's the same number of counts as your inhale. This would be 5/5/10/5. Practice walking while breathing in these ratios to increase the burning of fats without the damaging effects of a high heart rate.

Meditate on the choices that have brought you to this point. Make corrections, if applicable.

Repeat Day 17's technique, but reverse the sequence. Today inhale in four parts (quarters), and exhale in two parts (50/50). Notice the different qualities. This is a great practice for getting energized before a workout or a hike or before a morning business meeting.

P   Fully engage in the process of turning the breathing muscles on and off.

I   Each time we pause the breath, we're in meditation and mindfulness.

E   Emotions that distracted us from our intentions in the past are bypassed by the mind.

S   Creating space where there was previously no space or stressed awareness is fundamental to personal growth programming.

Today's Practice Notes

_____

_____

_____

_____

Day 19

*"You are the sum total of everything you've ever seen,
heard, eaten, smelled, been told, forgot—it's all there.
Everything influences each of us, and because of that
I try to make sure that my experiences are positive."*

— MAYA ANGELOU

OUR PERSONALITIES ARE SUCH A MINUTE aspect of who we truly are, but when they're in conflict with our soul, they can create great suffering. The suffering continues until we release our attachments to who we think we are and open ourselves to our true essence—pure consciousness.

For centuries, philosophers and curious people have pondered the questions: *Who am I?; Why am I here?; Where did I come from?; Where will I go?* Our answers to these questions give us clues about our life's purpose. Personalities provide a narrow view of traits and capabilities, but giving thought to these four questions expands our view of others and ourselves. The soul has the answers, but hearing them may mean delving a little bit deeper into each question. Breathe slowly and listen for your intuition and you'll hear the answers come from a place slightly deeper inside than where you were a moment ago. Smile and know you're safe.

Today's Practice

Repeat Day 18's technique, but reverse the sequence of the increments. Today inhale in thirds and exhale 50/50. Notice the different qualities of both. This is a great way to wake up and raise your energy level for physical and mental tasks.

Notice how quickly the breathing can take you deep inside. It's a highly efficient way to bypass the fear-centered lower ego and tune in to Source.

119

Sit with compassion and the courage to ask yourself the bigger questions about your life rather than focusing on the familiar old answers. Remain open and try not to expect the answer right away. Sometimes it's not about the answers but asking the right questions.

P Changing the fractions of inhale and exhale is perfect for the morning, before you work out or go to work.

I Notice the refinement of all your mental qualities of inhale, such as clearer thoughts. Notice the qualities of the exhale, amplifying the process of cleansing emotions without the dangers of a higher heart rate.

E Notice energy disguised as emotions and feelings moving through every cell in your body. Witness this process of transformation mindfully.

S Turning demonic to divine, evolving, and growing into a superior woman or man—this is your quest for the rest of your life. The key is to stay open. Open the chest, and relax the shoulders and arms when you walk.

Today's Practice Notes

Day 20

*"Breath control techniques are simple, effective ways
to stimulate and activate the vagus nerve. There are
whole new fields of medicine coming from the brain gut
connection. Part of life is about self care, caring for yourself
is the first step to caring about others. You can't care fully
about others, or for others if you're sick and dying."*

— ED HARROLD

T HE VAGUS NERVE IS LARGELY RESPONSIBLE for the mind-body connection, since it goes to all your major organs (except your adrenals and thyroid). It's intimately tied to how we connect with one another—it links directly to nerves that tune our ears to human speech, coordinate eye contact, and regulate emotional expressions. It also influences the release of oxytocin, a hormone that's important in social bonding.

The vagus nerve plays a huge role in our overall health. It's the main nerve involved in our immune system, the tenth cranial nerve, and the longest nerve in the body. The twelve cranial nerves are affected substantially by breathing through your nostrils. The vagus nerve runs from the brain through the center of the upper torso, through the diaphragm muscle and into the organs of the abdomen. It has jellyfish-type tentacles that connect with every digestive organ of the abdomen except for the adrenal glands. It's called the wandering nerve because of its length, and it's called the nerve of compassion because it can stimulate the release of calming serotonin when we're stressed. The vagus nerve lowers heart rate and blood pressure and stimulates digestion.

Strengthening the charge of energy that travels through the vagus nerve is one of the most effective ways to stall degenerative diseases. Learning pranayama is the fastest way to increase the charge of energy currents of the vagus nerve and receive the health benefits. The autonomic nervous system, which controls breath rates, energy usage, and brainwave activity, can then create a rejuvenating, peaceful body/mind state by rebuilding and strengthening the parasympathetic branch of the ANS.

The vagus nerve is the major nerve in the brain and body to help us breathe because it releases the neurotransmitter acetylcholine, which prevents inflammation and helps the brain make memories. When we're talking about cardiac health, the vagus nerve slows the pulse down, saving the heart from extra work.

As you strengthen the vagal pathway, everything in the body performs its functions with less stress on the system. There is less fear in our thinking and feeling about our life. As we relax, answers to lifelong challenges appear out of nowhere. The new science that's coming to us is promising for a more peaceful planet and species. All we need to do is apply it in our daily lives through conscious awareness and making mindful choices.

❋ *Today's Practice*

You're twenty days into your new breathing experiences, so review the past nineteen days and choose the practice you want to do today. By now, I'm sure many amazing things are starting to happen to your body and your thoughts and emotions. All yogic breathing stimulates vagal tone and parasympathetic strength. Meditate on which one you would like to experience.

Meditate on the space between the center of your brain and a space behind and below your navel. Witness the energy moving, and notice where you sense that the energy is stuck.

Remember, no more mouth breathing ever in your life. When you incorporate the pranayama breathing exercises, "Less is more" can be the bedrock of your personal awareness.

P Follow the diaphragm muscle downward on the inhale to a point behind your navel. Follow the exhale up the spine to a point in the center of your brain.

I Feel and relax your mind while you trace the energy of your breath from the belly to the brain. It's a north/south visualization.

E Imagine each breath is polishing the vertebra in your spine like fine pearls.

S Notice after several rounds how light you feel and how lighthearted you've become in a very short period of time.

Today's Practice Notes

_____

_____

_____

_____

Day 21

*"There is one way of breathing that is shameful and
constricted. Then, there's another way: a breath
of love that takes you all the way to infinity."*

— RUMI

ONE OF MY FIRST GOALS WITH CLIENTS is to correct their
breathing. As they strengthen their respiratory system,
they take a lot of unhealthy pressure off their heart. As their
breathing improves, so does their gastric fire from digestion
and assimilation. As this occurs, their blood pressure and
heart rate stabilize, the pace of their thoughts slows down,
and, in turn, they have less stress. Skillful breathing is where
the work begins.

The body basically works on pressure. Some pressure is
healthy, and some pressure is unhealthy, shortening the life span
of our cells. When unhealthy workloads are placed on the body,
acidity, phlegm, and toxins begin to poison the bloodstream,
making the heart muscle work harder and harder, leading to
exhaustion. When we're tired, it's hard—we can't pay attention
and be fully present.

As we apply the yogic breathing models, the body immediately begins the process of detoxification. When the body gets
happy, we feel better. When we feel good, our mind thinks good
thoughts. As respiratory muscles become stronger, we bring
more oxygen into our bodies, and that builds our inner fire.
When our fire is high with a resting heart rate, we can't help
but feel great about life. Practice breathing every day—it's the
first thing you did when you entered this world, and it will be
the last thing you do before you leave.

✴ *Today's Practice*

Quarters:

25 percent inhale

Pause

25 percent inhale

Pause

25 percent inhale

Pause

25 percent inhale

Pause

Repeat on exhales

Breathing with an ocean-sound breath, inhale and fill your lungs in 25 percent increments until they're filled without straining. Then hold. Exhale in 25 percent increments and pause for a moment. Repeat for five to fifteen minutes while seated or walking.

Meditate on keeping your breathing as smooth as possible.

This is an important note to the practitioner: The greater the space between the holdings, the more meditative it will become. This is also great for endurance athletes. In other words, the longer the holding times or pausing, the greater the meditation and transformation opportunities. Longer pauses are great, but don't put a strain on your breathing. Keep the breathing pace slow and under control. Once you master this while seated, try it walking, running, biking, or hiking. You will feel major shifts in your cardio workouts, without wear and tear to joints, muscles, and bones.

P Notice what happens physically when you turn the breathing muscles on and off.

I Notice the mental space between each little breath in and out.

E Be aware of the emotional spaces that are created while practicing this technique.

S Meditate on the highest good for yourself first and everyone else in your life second in every moment of your life. Put yourself first!

Today's Practice Notes

Day 22

"We live in an ocean of air like fish in a body of water. By our breathing we are attuned to our atmosphere. If we inhibit our breathing we isolate ourselves from the medium in which we exist. In all Oriental and mystic philosophies, the breath holds the secret to the highest bliss."

— ALEXANDER LOWEN

A TTUNING YOUR BODY TO THE SEASONS of the year is important to maximizing the benefits of Mother Nature's bounty and our connection with it. The four seasons produce different qualities that align with our internal cycles. How we interact with ourselves, how we care for ourselves on every level, should shift subtly but consciously with the seasons.

The fire/solar energy of spring and summer produce warm, humid air, and the body responds favorably to the warming quality. Moving the body becomes easier, the imagination begins to stir, and the abundance of sunlight helps to lift and stabilize our moods. The foods we eat are lighter, cooling, and easy to digest. With this lightness and warm air, we have extra energy available, and the season's solar light and elemental fires help the body to move blocked energy with more ease.

Autumn and winter produce the qualities of cool, dry, and the body may not do as well physically. Everything is a little arthritic and takes time to warm up. With the arthritic body comes the arthritic mind; creativity is stalled and there's little imagination. The foods of autumn and winter are more complex and warm, heavy, moist, and grounding, and take longer to digest. Energy levels may be low, with little sunlight and outdoor activity. It's a time of rest and introspection, but we still need to exercise every day to keep our energy high and moving through our body.

Learn about the strengths and challenges offered by the turning of the seasons, and remain mindful of these changes when planning your goals and transitions throughout a calendar year. Playing to the strengths of the qualities of the seasons puts us in a better position for success over the course of time.

☀ Today's Practice

Slow your breath and relax. Feel the current season's nature moving around you and within you. Begin the four-part breath. If it's spring or summer, exhale longer and hold the breath out a bit longer. This will cool your inner fires. If it's autumn or winter, increase the inhale and holding the breath in. This will create more fire.

EXAMPLE:

Spring/summer, 5/5/10/5 or 5/5/5/10. This is cooling balance.

Autumn/winter, 8/16/8/8, or 8/24/8/8. This is warming balance.

P Feel the breath being turned on and off until your lungs are full or empty. This rise and fall of energy is the foundation of a balanced day.

I Begin to see that the mind is your best friend, not your enemy. When you fight with your mind, you fight with yourself.

E No one has become successful from activating negativity or negative emotions. When emotions are cooled, old fears turn into new strengths.

S Breathing with longer external retentions activates a deeper trust. We trust that everything has
a deeper meaning, that there aren't any mistakes,
only lessons.

Today's Practice Notes

Day 23

*"No problem will be solved at the same level
of consciousness it was created."*

— ALBERT EINSTEIN

T HIS QUOTE CHANGED MY LIFE FOREVER. Einstein's famous statement can be helpful when applied to conscious communication with others and ourselves. Einstein was very spiritual. He didn't dare let on about this early in his career, as he would have been an outcast and not taken seriously by the conservative scientific community of his day. But as he aged, his quotes became sage-like, almost mystical. He was not only an intellectual genius with extraordinary cognitive ability but a very wise man who deeply understood the importance of consciousness and began unraveling the workings of the Universe itself.

Our conscious thoughts become words and actions, so we want to be as informed as possible. We are beings of light, all light is energy and so, in essence, we are energy.

High-frequency energy waves have more peaks and troughs within an established distance and therefore contain more information than lower-frequency waves, which have fewer peaks and troughs in the same distance and carry less information. When we meditate, we lower our vibration, which helps the mind to become still and quiet. There are fewer information waves streaming through our brain and body when we switch from high beta brain wave states into low alpha brain waves and toward Zen. From this grounded, centered place, we can use pranayama or guided mindfulness to raise our frequency and open to more universal guidance and information. When we're well informed, we make healthier choices and feel more at peace.

✳ *Today's Practice*

Alternate Nostril Breathing with Internal and External Holdings:

Today's practice is the same as Day 16, except we now add a holding-out period after the end of an exhale.

For today's practice, you'll need to slow down and pay attention to details or you may get lost in the meditative mind quickly while you hold your breath out.

Start by closing off the right nostril and using ocean-sound breath. Slowly inhale up the left nasal channel, hold the breath for a moment, close off the left nasal channel, release the right thumb and exhale out the right nasal channel. Pause and hold breath out for a moment. Inhale up the right nasal channel and hold breath in. Close the right nasal channel, release your ring finger and exhale out the left nasal channel. Pause and hold breath out. Repeat for five to fifteen minutes and then meditate.

P Notice how quickly this practice positively affects your nervous system. That old dried-out, fried nervous system is now moist, lubricated, and repaired. The more alkaline your body is, the lower your acidity and the less inflammation you have.

I There isn't any thought pattern or part of the mind that you can't analyze or reflect on for longer than you could twenty-three days ago.

E Perceptions of old emotions or events from our past might now have a different story. Keep feeling this refined awareness of your emotional content.

S   There are only lessons. Failure doesn't exist. Stay light; don't get too heavy on any level.

Today's Practice Notes

_____

_____

_____

_____

Day 24

"For breath is life, and if you breathe
well you will live long on earth."

— SANSKRIT PROVERB

ACCORDING TO AYURVEDA, doing a cleanse twice a year is very helpful in removing excess wastes from the digestive tract and toxins from the cellular body. Plan a cleanse for spring and autumn—they're the perfect times to rest, repair, and restore the body.

Removing excess mucus and undigested wastes from the body is a great way to stay young and stall the aging process. Dr. Richard Anderson is the American father of cleansing, and I've used his product, Arise and Shine, for many years to clean my organs and clear my mind. Dr. Anderson calls the excessive waste that's removed from the digestive organs "mucoid plaque." When this plaque builds up on the internal walls of the colon, it takes a lot of extra energy to push our food through and out of the body. We only have so much energy each day, and when most of our energy is used to remove dirty water, toxins, and mucus, that leaves little energy for the brain. When the colon is cleared, all the energy we used to use to digest can be diverted to our brain, our blood is purified of toxins, and oxygen flows through our arteries to our organs and systems without impediment.

When we cleanse our body, we also cleanse our mind. The mind becomes like a laser in its new awareness, clear and coherent. We can become so crystal clear it can be daunting; our senses are heightened, and gathering insights and information becomes effortless. Our perception of life itself changes and expands into unlimited potential and a deep understanding of our connection to all things.

Today's Practice

Agni Sara, or washing the energy centers of the abdomen:

Sitting or standing, slow down your breathing and straighten your spine. Become aware of the abdominal muscles from your navel to your solar plexus. Slowly inhale to 75 percent of your lungs' capacity. While holding the breath in, rhythmically pump your upper abdominal muscles out and in. This raises energy quickly and clears the four upper organs of the abdomen. Exhale slowly and completely through your nose.

Practice this on an empty stomach. Try to pump the belly muscles first slowly, and then pick up the pace to one round per second. This is fantastic in the early-morning hours for igniting the inner fires before we start the day's activities. It's the perfect warm-up on every level. Start with ten to twenty rounds and build up quickly to seventy-five to one hundred.

P Pushing oxygen molecules deeper into your nervous system and tissues provides a big advantage to your overall energy levels. It helps hydrogen to keep cells healthy and alkalized.

I Handling more and more energy in the mind will raise your personal awareness overnight. This builds self-esteem and confidence.

E Most people can't control their feelings, and this gets us in trouble. Feelings come from the gut, so removing toxic material from the intestines gets us in touch with our gut intuition.

S As we replace unhealthy competition (I'm better, you're better) with healthy compassion, we remember that everyone is working on something and doing the best they can at their level of awareness.

Today's Practice Notes

Day 25

*"Whenever you have a spare moment in life,
scan your eyes and low jaw area and deeply
relax these areas again and again."*

— ED HARROLD

THERE ARE THREE PLACES IN MY BODY where I tend to hold stress: my hands, feet, and face. All of these are uniquely connected to my solar plexus and my personal power.

Our facial expressions reflect how we really feel about something or someone. The muscles around the eyes and lower jaw are connected deeply to our belly and specifically to our solar plexus. When we strain our facial features, we create blocked energy or stress in the belly and we don't feel as powerful or confident. The face and belly automatically sense our hands and evaluate whether the fist is clenched or the fingers are relaxed. The feet let our brains know whether we're in or out of balance. The somatic nervous system does all this to protect us.

Today's Practice

Deeply massage your feet with oil to keep them moist and flexible and to provide you with awareness and balance from the ground up. Stretch your fingers and massage your hands, keeping the energy moving and removing stiffness from your joints. Massage your temples, allowing you to focus and slow your thought. Mindful compassionate massage releases endorphins and serotonin in the body, bringing you into a state of healing and calmness. Throughout the day, remind yourself to relax your lower jaw and the muscles that move your eyes. The yoga posture called the "Lion's Pose" is great for releasing tension from the face and the brain. This helps your stress levels significantly, and you'll sleep better at night. Practice the Lion's Pose daily and massage your feet, hands, and temples a few times a week.

Today's breathing practice is the same as Day 24's except we will do the agni sara with breath held out after the exhale.

Start with ten to twenty rounds and build to seventy-five to one hundred.

P   Go slowly and build up fire. As abdominal nerve endings that control the belly are energized, we become more aware of the role of the body.

I   Pay attention to the mind after you complete the technique and your energy settles. You will notice a sharper, clearer mind.

E   "Washing" the stomach—clearing out the mucus, fats, and phlegm—is the physical goal of today's practice. Emotions live in the gut, and this exercise will clean out old emotional content. It's like taking the trash out.

S   When the inside of your belly is clean, your heart, which is the master of all feelings and emotions, begins to take control of your life.

Today's Practice Notes

Day 26

*"When the breath wanders the mind also is unsteady.
But when the breath is calmed the mind too will
be still, and the yogi achieves long life. Therefore,
one should learn to control the breath."*

— SVATMARAMA, "HATHA PRADIPIKA"

THE GREAT THING ABOUT LIFE IS THAT we get to re-create ourselves every day. Every single day is a new opportunity, a time to shed our past, whether we perceive it as good or bad. Every sunrise is new experience entirely; it's different from the day before. When we look at life through this lens, we see that each new second is a fresh opportunity and we're less likely to get stuck in depression or noncreative states.

The Greek philosopher Heraclitus said, "No man ever steps in the same river twice, for it's not the same river and he's not the same man." The only constant in our lives is change. Life flows forward and so do we. Events rarely play out the same way twice. Let's say you have a party at your house, friends come over, and you have a magnificent time. You say to yourself, let's have another party and invite the same people over and have the same wine and food—it'll be great. You may still have a wonderful time but can't help noticing that the second party isn't the same as the first. Something or many things were different. Every moment of our life is a completely fresh experience happening only one time. The ego is so afraid of this phenomenon that it scares us into thinking we have to replay a past event to be safe. That's fear-based thinking, and it's the opposite of what's true.

When we came out of the womb, every moment was fresh and new, and we were completely in the present moment. Past and future didn't exist. This doesn't change as we age; it stays the same for our whole life. The heart is always in the present, keeping you alive. It's the head that's replaying a past event, wishing to change it or deny it, or future tripping about what might happen tomorrow. Use your breath, connect with your heart, and create the moment you deserve. You deserve the best—always have, always will.

✳ Today's Practice

Practice Day 10 again today. After the breathing exercise, silently chant, "I am light in action," for as long as you desire.

P Use a slower inhale and exhale to become more and more present. Sense a lighter version of yourself moving through you and rising to the surface.

I Stay present for the shifts in the mind and the new perceptions of old thought forms.

E Cooling emotions and then heating them up is the practice today. Notice how you feel afterward.

S Most of us come to spiritual practice after everything else has failed. That's okay—it's all part of your plan to heal your life, learn your lessons, get up on the medal podium again, and stay there.

Today's Practice Notes

_____

_____

_____

_____

Day 27

*"Our body has this defect that,
the more it is provided care and comforts,
the more needs and desires it finds."*

— SAINT TERESA OF AVILA

IF YOU WANT TO CHANGE YOUR LIFE, one of the great tools is nutrition. The nervous system responds to the frequency of the nutrients we eat. The classic western diet that most of us grew up on is toxic and acidic. This makes it very hard on the body to remove the toxins in our environment and keeps us stuck in the old programming. There are many crash-and-fad diets out there, but remember the first three letters of diet are DIE.

Most nutritionists agree that alkalizing our tissues by eating lighter nutritional sources is a must. The foods in the typical American diet are very acidic and form mucus when we don't quickly burn them for fuel.

This mucus is like quicksand to our creativity and intuition; we're easily depressed, hard on ourselves, and feel negative about our life's efforts and the efforts of others.

When we eat what's fresh, local, and in season and what our body is calling for, which is often different than what our head wants, we begin to change how we perceive not just our nutrition, but life itself. We make choices based on our perceptions and our choices create our consequences. Eat only what the body calls for to fuel itself and control your portion size and the time of day you eat to suit your individual constitution.

⚜ *Today's Practice*

Practice gentle pranayama before, during, and after your meals. Get centered before the meal and breathe slowly during the meal. Don't rush the energy into the body. After you eat, go for a short walk and consciously breathe. When it's possible, take an eight- to fifteen-minute nap after the walk to help your body with the DEA process: digestion, elimination, assimilation. When you can, lie on your left side for ten minutes after you wake from the nap and meditate deeply on your body's needs for energy and a clean, light diet. The head usually hijacks the body's needs and the body suffers. Practice noticing when your body is asking for nutrients and how your ego mentally shifts that. Sometimes a piece of pizza is exactly what the body needs. Sometimes the ego will say to you, *If one piece is this good we should have two or three more.* Sometimes a burger is just the type of grounding food we need, but not two or three burgers. This type of emotional eating is dangerous. Keep a keen eye on your portions and have a lot of many different types of food on your plate.

P   Silently repeat the phrase "soft belly."

I   Mentally "witness" the internal. Ask "What does my body really require right now?"

E   Let all emotions have a *temporary pass.* Just let them move through you without comparison, labels, or judgments.

S   We can't master the mind without cooperation of the gut and the microbiome of the gut; this is key.

Today's Practice Notes

_____

_____

_____

_____

Day 28

"It is by going down into the abyss that
we recover the treasures of life. Where you
stumble, there lies your treasure."

— JOSEPH CAMPBELL

MOTHER NATURE IS SUCH A GREAT TEACHER. She shows us the interconnectedness of all living things. It's a reminder of how much is expected of us. We have to work hard without attachment to the outcome. We all suffer on this planet; it's how we respond to the suffering that makes our life or breaks it.

Nature is our mirror and our timeless teacher. When our ego and attachments shrink us, Mother Nature stretches us and expands us to our humanness. Have you ever seen an uprooted tree? The entwined circle of roots looks like an art sculpture. The real beauty of the tree isn't only what's above ground; it's also what's below. This is how life really is. We all need each other. We are one and there is no true separation between us. Just as the roots, dirt, soil, rain, and sunlight is required for a tree to grow and survive, we need each other and this Earth to truly thrive. There is so much going on underneath the surface of it all to give the bounty of the visual on the surface. There is always more than meets the eye.

The way back to self begins with letting go of all thought forms and belief systems that separate us from all that is; separation with self, separation with others and even with the planet. We can be alone without being lonely and also find comfort in the truth that we are never truly alone. We are fully supported and loved at all times; love is an inside job. Now take a look at how you share love and contribute to the world. Figure out if what you do for a living, what you want to do, is in alignment with your values and who you want to be as a person. This is an acquired skill and takes time. There will be errors in judgment along the way as we can only make choices based on the information we have in the moment. The more understanding we gain through direct experience, the more informed we become. This allows us to make better choices that reinforce our values and intentions for living.

When we fall or create deep misalignment in our lives, immediately asking two questions helps bring us into mindfulness and accountability, setting us up for transformation and growth. The first question is, "How did I fall?" The second is, "How fast can I get back up, while integrating the wisdom of life's experience, accepting that even difficult challenges and upsets have value?"

Allow Mother Nature to show you the big picture and her beauty any time you have fallen or feel alone in an unhealthy way. She will breathe life back into you where you need it most in that moment. Remember, she honors and accepts all of you and supports you on your journey. Mother Earth provides everything you need to live and sustain yourself. Begin a conscious relationship of gratitude with her. As you acknowledge her grace and abundance you may find yourself opening to trust and knowing that you are truly provided for.

❄ *Today's Practice*

Do fifty rounds of power breathing and then meditate on the breath for a few moments.

Power breathing is done by taking a passive inhale at a moderate or gentle pace through the nostrils and an active, forceful exhalation out the nose by pulling the solar plexus and abdomen in toward the spine quickly and rapidly following with a completely passive inhalation. Find a steady rhythm to the movement doing one round per second and feel your belly pumping the air out through your nostrils. Try to keep facial muscles relaxed during this breathing exercise.

Continue with another fifty rounds, this time with a slightly slower pace, and then meditate for a few minutes

Continue for another fifty rounds, breathing as fast as possible, and then meditate for as long as time allows. Look and listen deeply inside for guidance.

As you develop more healthy control inside yourself, you'll experience more healthy control in your relationships.

P   Imagine you're breathing with the earth, as one with the earth, no separation, no fragmentation. Start today's technique slowly and try to find a rhythm to the pace. After you master the technique over several weeks, try to build up the speed of the in-and-out breath.

I   What you see outside of you is a reflection of some seed inside looking for wholeness. This practice clears the neural circuits and feedback loops between the brain and the heart.

E   Fully feel each breath in and out without straining. Feel how everything is in balance in nature. Winter/summer, sunrise/sunset, everything is always searching for balance.

S   Learn to be "open" for longer and longer. Through your five sensors—eyes, ears, nose, mouth, and the sense of touch—feel the interconnectedness of everything around you and in you right now. The breath is very transformational and accelerates our growth beyond our lower ego. Less is sometimes more in life.

Today's Practice Notes

Day 29

"Unworthiness is the inmost frightening thought that you do not belong, no matter how much you want to belong, that you are an outsider and will always be an outsider. It is the idea that you are flawed and cannot be fixed. It is wanting to be loved and feeling unlovable, or wanting to love and feeling that you are not capable of loving."

— GARY ZUKAV

WE SPEND SO MUCH OF OUR precious life looking for something of value *out there*. That puts a lot of pressure on us to become something we equate or define as valuable externally, complete with an impressive title and status. We begin the never-ending struggle to "keep up with the Joneses." Now, more than ever, we need to resist that temptation. Looking inward first is the key to a healthy mental outlook of life's external gifts.

If we were fortunate enough to have a safe and loving childhood we only concerned ourselves with the present moment. That moment was grounded with inward focus first. As time went by, between the ages of five and ten, we began to look outward and discovered that we were each unique, there were others out there different than each of us. We met people who dressed differently than we did, talked differently, and liked different foods, scents, and colors. This was our first opportunity to start seeing strength in diversity. We all aren't the same on the outside, but we are on the inside. We began to give away our internal power when we compared ourselves with others and thought they were better than us and thought our lives would be better if we were someone else. The problem with that is that you were born to be uniquely you.

The Yogic path refers to this as attachment and says it's the root cause of all suffering. Looking outside yourself wanting more, or thinking you're better or worse than others is a waste of time. Life is about the inner journey. Connect yourself to your inner strengths. Let those inner strengths guide you through the illusion world outside of us where we think we need a material thing, or we think we should be more like someone else. There isn't anyone out there that's better than you and there isn't anyone out there that's worse than you. We're all equal and nonseparate. It's just you and God having a conversation in a physical, feeling body, on a planet out in space called Earth. Breathe into your inner space today and fill it with God's voice, the conscious collective inside of you.

⚹⚹ Today's Practice

Today we'll practice ocean-sound breathing while we inhale in sixths and exhale in twelfths.

1. Inhale in six small inhales and hold breath for a few seconds.

2. Exhale slowly in twelve small exhales until your lungs are empty.

Repeat this sequence for five to fifteen minutes.

Notice what occurred to your perceptions when you doubled the small exhalations. Did you feel yourself calming, relaxing, and softening?

Our minds usually describe time to us in a contracted way and that doesn't leave space for joy. We always seem rushed in life. Slow your breathing down and feel an expansion in your sense of time. Live from your heart, it's always right on time.

Our thoughts dictate an emotional response, which we feel in the body. Draw strength from your heart as you learn to *feel* uncomfortable emotions instead of pushing them away. Breathe into this process, calm your emotions, and get out of your own way. Let it happen again and again. *Go be great!*

P   Relax your facial area completely, sense your heartbeat, and visualize breathing in and out through your heart only.

I   Sit in your inner mind and observe the process of life without judgment.

E   Relax your belly. Emotional wisdom is now key in your life and how you're showing up in your life.

S   Keep softening when there's the opportunity. Soften in and around what was hard or too stiff to communicate with in the past. Keep softening; this is true strength.

Today's Practice Notes

_____

_____

_____

_____

Day 30

*"The nose is for breathing,
the mouth is for eating."*

— PROVERB

NOSTRIL BREATHING IS THE MAJOR KEY for transformation. Transformation requires us to become aware of an internal flow of emotions (energy) with an intention (self-awareness) for daily incremental personal and professional improvement. Emotions become the framework of our internal growth. The trick is in knowing that our old fears are disguised as new strengths.

Compassionate leaders have strong internal mapping processes that lead to an equal exchange of energy in all relationships. When energy is exchanged equally in our personal and professional life, we incur no karma from the interactions. This is a physical, mental, emotional, and spiritual quest for your best. Go *be* great. Allow the power of the heart to fuel the brain and fire the mind into *greatness*. Breathe into your heart space to correctly set this formula in motion.

⋇ *Today's Practice*

Using Ocean-Sound Breath:

1. Make your exhales longer than your inhales for several moments.

2. Practice four-part breath with emphasis on holding the breath in.

   (i.e., Inhale for six/hold for eigtheen/exhale for six. Repeat this seven to ten times

3. Practice fractal breathing, inhaling in one-sevenths and exhaling in one-fourteenths. Repeat this seven to ten times

4. Practice agni sara. (If you want a refresher, see Day 24.)

5. Practice power breathing for one hundred rounds; *one-third regular pace, one-third slower pace, and one-third faster pace.* Exhale all the air and hold your breath out and count. Then, inhale, hold in twice the count you're holding out. For example, if you're holding out for ten counts, hold in for twenty counts.

6. Practice alternate nostril breathing for seven to ten rounds.

7. Meditate on your journey, on all the information you have become aware of in this book. Know that this is just the start. The universe sees you and hears you and must help you when you ask.

P   My heart is fearless. Every slow breath is searching for buried treasure inside me and bringing
it to the surface of my mind.

I   My past is a plus. Everything in my life is happening for my benefit.

E   I love my emotions. My emotions love me.

S   Today is the day. Every day is my day. I am my
days, my days aren't me.

Today's Practice Notes

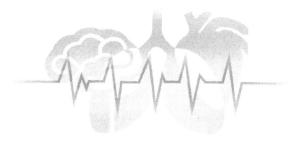

Optimum Health Through Breath

"The goal of life is to make your heartbeat match the beat of the universe, to match your nature with Nature."

— Joseph Campbell

OPTIMAL HEALTH IS MUCH MORE attainable than you've been led to believe. It doesn't take long hours of training, and you don't have to push yourself to the point of exhaustion when you work out. That doesn't mean there won't be times to push a little, but if you're pushing so hard that you need to breathe through your mouth, you're doing more harm than good in the long run. And life itself is a long run. If life's a race, it's a race to come in last, not first. So take your time. Life has little intervals of speed, but predominantly it's an endurance event.

Everything I've shared in this book, I've been practicing myself for years. I love the science, but what I love more is that

I'm in better shape physically, mentally, and emotionally today than I was when I was half this age.

To give you an example of how this plays out in my life, about five years ago I met with a team of technicians at a health and wellness company called CardioKinetics to take its stress test and show them what conscious breathing can do in a high-heart-rate activity. (I should mention I forgot to bring exercise clothes and sneakers, so I did this test in slacks and bare feet!) It was a treadmill test with uphill sections and downhill sections, and I have no idea how long it lasted. Throughout the test, I used various nostril-breathing techniques to keep my heart rate down for as long as possible. At some point I could see on the monitors that my heart rate was starting to rise, and I could feel the resistance building.

When the technician stopped the test, my heart rate was at 185 and I was still breathing through my nose. He said he'd never seen anyone complete the test without breathing through their mouth. "We don't even have a score for someone fifty-one years old that performed like you just did," he said after reading the printout of the report. "You scored in the top one percentile for a twenty-year-old male."

But what really blew his mind was that after I stepped off the treadmill with a heart rate of 185, it took only thirty seconds for it drop to 135. If I'd been breathing through my mouth, it would have taken fifteen to twenty minutes to drop to 135. Larger amounts of cooling parasympathetic hormones were in my system because I was breathing diaphragmatically and stimulating my vagus nerve. Mouth-breathers will take minutes to get their heart rate down rather than seconds, and they have very low vagal tone. Hence, heart disease is the leading cause of death in the world, even among athletes.

I attribute the majority of my good health and well-being to the breathing practices I've included in this book, which I do daily. No matter what area of life or domain you want to excel in, you've just taken the first step by reading this book and doing the practices. We have to retrain the body and mind to operate from a balanced autonomic nervous system, and hopefully you've seen for yourself by now that the retraining begins and ends with your breath. The fact that breathing is the only involuntary body function we can directly and consciously control is not a fluke or a coincidence. We were given the controls to this system so that we can enjoy a long healthy life. Science has confirmed what yogis have known for centuries: controlling our breathing can slow our heart rate, which ultimately extends our lives. So if you're searching for a fountain of youth, deepen your inhale, lengthen your exhale and slow the pace at which you do both.

From a scientific perspective, amplifying the effects of strengthening the abdominal diaphragm muscle and the qualities of the vagus nerve through the breathing techniques in this book are an unbeatable combination. Every cell and system of your body benefits, including the brain. This unique combination of increasing the strength and range of motion of the diaphragm muscle and amplifying the route and current of the vagus nerve makes this one of the ultimate ways to increase mental energy levels and also calm every system in the body, stalling aging.

My hope is that through this book you've discovered the fundamentals of living your life with breath. By incorporating a daily practice for yourself, you will continue to enjoy the same discoveries I'm still enjoying on a regular basis with myself and my clients.

Be patient. This is a process. At the beginning and end of each day, carve out some time for these techniques. Start the practices from Day 1 and continue until you've completed all thirty days. After that, you can repeat the program in the same order or skip around to meet your own needs and desires. *The secret is to commit to daily practice for a year.* By the end of the year, your nervous system will have learned new patterns, your brain will have created new feedback loops and conscious breathing will have become a way of life.

Remember that every day you have a choice, a choice to grow or shrink. We grow when we move beyond that internal negative voice that's creating distraction or saying, "You don't have time to do your breathing practice today." I try to stay open all the time—opening my chest and relaxing my shoulders and arms. I stay open for one breath longer than yesterday. I don't shut down communication; I prefer to be fearless and relaxed. For most of us, it's an incremental process of daily growth without ego attachments. When we're open, life is as good as it gets. Open can be the opposite of closed down and stressed out as a result of old, outdated thoughts and feelings. Or open can just mean "I'm open." That's it. Notice your overall feeling when you're open; it's a combination of deep listening and a calm but powerful sense of self.

The proven benefits of conscious breathing are based on simple science:

1. The fewer breaths you take per minute, the lower your heart rate and blood pressure.

2. With the lower heart rate, your thoughts will be more organized, and when you're stressed you can quickly restore a mental state of balance.

3. When your brain's fear centers don't sense danger, your brain tells your body to burn its fat stores instead of your precious sugar supplies.

4. As the mind-body science shows, conscious breathing improves the ability to accomplish any type of task.

5. Strengthening the diaphragm muscle enables optimal breathing and digestion, which leads to improved brain power and better choices.

Emotional intelligence is our ability to feel anything and everything and, in the moment, to thoughtfully consider and choose what to do or say in response. It's a learned practice, and the learning curve can be shortened considerably with conscious, pranayama breathing.

As we connect with feeling centers in our nerve endings, our mental and emotional intelligence evolves in two ways:

1. Feeling our thoughts for longer with a mindful breath gives us valuable insight into what's really in front of us right now, in this moment. Feel thoughts, feel thoughts— this is the 101 level of self-improvement, without ego attachment to outcomes. The concept of winners and losers is irrelevant.

2. Using the body and breath as a source of intelligence, we can stay mentally balanced longer today than yesterday. The body feels our mental choices, and the sensations we experience are attempting to help us make the best choices possible. The brain loves when the body is involved in the choices it makes based on our perceptions.

The brain loves to read the whole landscape in the mind and body before choosing an action.

With the slower breath, we feel more and we begin to process more information without straining the mental processing centers of the left side of the prefrontal cortex, which contains our math and science application centers. The right prefrontal cortex is the arts and science department. There's a saying that you can't fix your mind with your mind. In other words, thoughts can't fix thoughts, because thoughts can't feel and so they don't think anything is wrong.

When you slow the breathing, it slows down time and we experience "now." The slower breathing activates a relaxation response; time is slowed down, thought is slowed down. And when our thoughts slow down, questions start to form around our old, time-tested answers. Adding the component of feeling moves us into the right prefrontal cortex and out of the time-based and thought-based left cortex.

We feel thoughts in our bodies before they register in our minds. This is classic Western neuroplasticity in action, folks. We can do this on demand any time we *slow down* our breath.

I hope you'll use the techniques in this book to help you grow beyond what you thought you could. The breath is a shortcut to processing our life and reorganizing it again and again. We will always want to know more; that's personal growth. The breath's growth model is inside-out growth, just like a seed. Once the seed develops into a plant or tree, it produces new seeds of its own, and those seeds take root and continue the cycle. The ability to control your inner environment empowers you to foster the atmosphere that guarantees a bountiful crop of creativity and new ideas every season. This learning cycle keeps us young in our hearts, and young and light in our minds.

Be your greatness. To be it, you *must* live it.

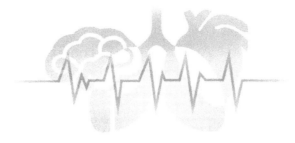

About the Author

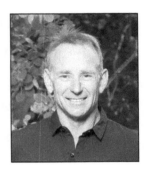

ED HARROLD is an inspirational leader, public speaker, coach, and educator. Ed's mastery in the science of mindful breathing has guided him to apply conscious breathing practices in corporate performance coaching, fitness and athletic training, healthcare trainings, stress reduction, and overall health and well-being.

Today, Ed blends the fields of neuroscience and the wisdom of contemplative traditions into effective strategies to improve well-being in Corporate America, healthcare, athletic performance, and individual health. Ed's fluency in mindfulness-based strategies, combined with the belief in the human potential, gives him the depth and understanding to meet individuals and group needs across industries and platforms.

Ed is a contributing health and wellness editor for HuffingtonPost, Thrive Global, MindBodyGreen, PTOnTheNet, and Corporate Wellness Magazine. Ed is on the Advisory Board for BreatheAware; a stress and resilience platform for individuals, employers, doctors, and coaches. Ed is an approved provider of Continuing Medical Education with George Washington University School of Medicine & Health Sciences as well as the American Council on Exercise. Experience Ed's MindBodyAthlete™, Executive Performance Coaching, Simplicity of Stress, and professional CME trainings nationally and internationally.

To continue your "life with breath", Ed is available for the following:

- Public Speaking Events

- Corporate Wellness Programs

- Corporate Leadership and Performance Coaching

- Individual Video Conferencing Sessions

- Fitness and Athletic Training for teams, trainers, and/ or individual athletes

- Health-care Trainings on using Breath AS Medicine

Learn more about Ed at *www.edharrold.com*

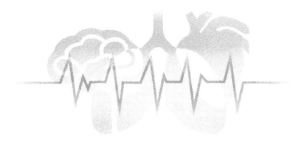

References

To learn the breathing techniques referenced in the 30-day plan, visit Ed Harrold's YouTube page *https://www.youtube.com/channel/ UCmYrluRdfY_Tw52C9MqlQxA*

[1] *New York Times*, "Breathe. Exhale. Repeat: The Benefits of Controlled Breathing," Nov. 9, 2016, *https://www.nytimes.com/2016/11/09/well/ mind/breathe-exhale-repeat-the-benefits-of-controlled-breathing. html?_r=1*

[2] Wu, W.J., S.H. Wang, W. Ling, L.J. Geng, X.X. Zhang, L. Yu, J. Chen, J.X. Luo and H.L. Zhao, 2017. Morning breathing exercises prolong lifespan by improving hyperventilation in people living with respiratory cancer. *Medicine* 96(2).

[3] Mahinrad, S., D. Van Heemst, P.W. Macfarlane, D.J. Stott, J.W. Jukema, A.J. De Craen and B.J. Sabayan, 2015. Short-term heart rate variability and cognitive function in older subjects at risk of cardiovascular disease. *Hypertension* 33, Suppl. 1.

[4] Jerath, R., J.W. Edry, V.A. Barnes and V. Jerath, 2006. Physiology of long pranayamic breathing: Neural respiratory elements may provide a mechanism that explains how slow deep breathing shifts the autonomic nervous system. *Medical Hypotheses* 67(3): 566–571.

[5] Pal, G.K., A. Agarwal, S. Karthik, P. Pal and N. Nanda, 2014. "Slow Yogic Breathing Through Right and Left Nostril Influences Sympathovagal Balance, Heart Rate Variability, and Cardiovascular Risks in Young Adults." *N Am J Med Sci.* 6(3): 145–151.

[6] Qu, S., S.M. Olafsrud, L.A. Meza-Zepeda and F. Saatcioglu, 2013. "Rapid Gene Expression Changes in Peripheral Blood Lymphocytes upon Practice of a Comprehensive Yoga Program," Ed. Srinivas Mummidi. *PLoS One* 8(4).

[7] Kox, M., L.T. van Eijk, J. Zwaag, J. van den Wildenberg, F.C.G.J. Sweep, J.G. van der Hoeven, and P. Pickkers, 2014. "Voluntary activation of the sympathetic nervous system and attenuation of the innate immune response in humans." Ed. Tamas L. Horvath. *Proc Natl Acad Sci USA* 111(20): 7379–7384.

[8] Bonaz, B., V. Sinniger and S. Pellissier, 2016. "Vagal tone: effects on sensitivity, motility, and inflammation." *Neurogastroenterol Motil* 28(4): 455–62.

[9] "When somebody loses weight, where does the fat go?" *BMJ* 2014;349:g7257

[10] Vera, F.M., J.M. Manzaneque, E.F. Maldonado, G.A. Carranque, F.M. Rodriguez, M.J. Blanca, M. Morell, 2009. "Subjective sleep quality and hormonal modulation in long-term yoga practitioners." *Biological Psychology* 81(3): 164–168.

[11] Khalsa, S.B., 2004. "Treatment of chronic insomnia with yoga: a preliminary study with sleep-wake diaries." *Appl Psychophysiol Biofeedback.* 29(4): 269–78.

[12] Bordoni, B., E. Zanier. "Anatomic connections of the diaphragm influence of respiration on the body system." *J Multidiscip Healthc* 2013, no. 6: 281–291.

[13] Djupesland, P.G., J.M. Chatkin, W. Qian and J.S. Haight, 2001. "Nitric oxide in the nasal airway: a new dimension in otorhinolaryngology." *Am J Otolaryngol* 22(1): 19–32.

[14] Sinicki, A., "The Neuroscience of Highly Productive Flow States," The Bioneer, *http://www.thebioneer.com/neuroscience-of-flow-states/*

[15] Elliott, S. "Diaphragm Mediates Action of Autonomic and Enteric Nervous Systems." *Psychophysiology* (Jan. 8, 2010).

Lightning Source UK Ltd.
Milton Keynes UK
UKHW020853230420
362135UK00016BA/375